IMAT Practice Papers

Volume One

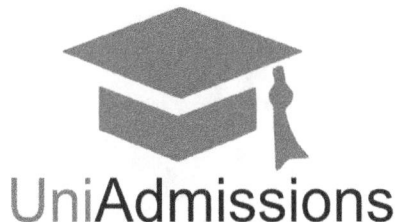

Copyright © 2019 *UniAdmissions*. All rights reserved.

ISBN 978-1-912557-79-0

No part of this publication may be reproduced or transmitted in any form or by any means, electronic or mechanical, including photocopying, recording, or by any information retrieval system without prior written permission of the publisher. This publication may not be used in conjunction with or to support any commercial undertaking without the prior written permission of the publisher.

Published by *RAR Medical Services Limited*
www.uniadmissions.co.it
info@uniadmissions.co.it
Tel: 0208 068 0438

This book is neither created nor endorsed by IMAT. The authors and publisher are not affiliated with IMAT. The information offered in this book is purely advisory and any advice given should be taken within this context. As such, the publishers and authors accept no liability whatsoever for the outcome of any applicant's IMAT performance, the outcome of any university applications or for any other loss. Although every precaution has been taken in the preparation of this book, the publisher and author assume no responsibility for errors or omissions of any kind. Neither is any liability assumed for damages resulting from the use of information contained herein. This does not affect your statutory rights.

IMAT Practice Papers
4 Full Papers & Solutions

Alex Ochakovski
Rohan Agarwal

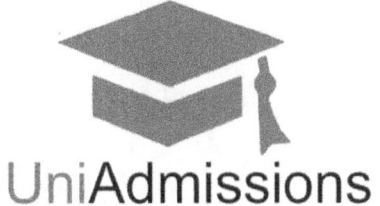

About the Authors

Alex is the co-founder and **Managing Director** at IMAT School, as well as the founder of MEDschool.it website. As a graduate of a first of a kind International Medical School in Italy, a former official supervisor of the IMAT test in Pavia and a dedicated curator of MEDschool.it, Alex has developed a deep understanding of the IMAT and the admission process over the years, following IMAT from the day it was created.

As an avid researcher with over ten peer-reviewed publications, experienced software developer, a fluent speaker of five languages and a medical doctor, Alex feels most fulfilled by combining his passions and strengths in projects that make a positive impact on society.

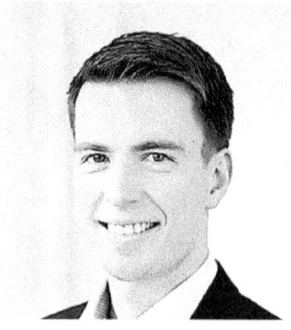

Thousands of current international medical students have been admitted to medical studies all over Italy with the help of the guidance and resources he provides to this day, creating a country-wide network of contacts in every International Medical School in Italy.

Rohan is the **Director of Operations** at *UniAdmissions* and is responsible for its technical and commercial arms. He graduated from Gonville and Caius College, Cambridge and is a fully qualified doctor. Over the last five years, he has tutored hundreds of successful Oxbridge and Medical applicants. He has also authored twenty books on admissions tests and interviews.

Rohan has taught physiology to undergraduate medical students and interviewed medical school applicants for Cambridge. He has published research on bone physiology and writes education articles for the Independent and Huffington Post. In his spare time, Rohan enjoys playing the piano and table tennis.

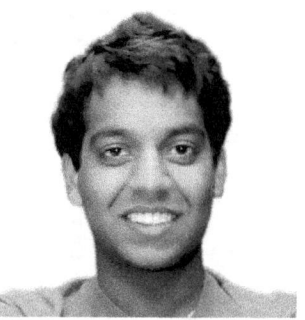

Introduction 6
General Advice 7
Revision Timetable 12
Getting the most out of Mock Papers 13
Things to have done before using this book 14
Section 1: An Overview 16
Sections 2, 3 & 4: An Overview 17
How to use this Book 18
Scoring Tables 19

Mock Paper A 21
Section 1 21
Section 2 25
Section 3 29
Section 4 31

Mock Paper B 33
Section 1 33
Section 2 38
Section 3 42
Section 4 44

Mock Paper C 46
Section 1 46
Section 2 51
Section 3 55
Section 4 58

Mock Paper D 60
Section 1 60
Section 2 64
Section 3 68
Section 4 71

Answer Key 75
Mock Paper A Answers 76
Mock Paper B Answers 82
Mock Paper C Answers 88
Mock Paper D Answers 97

INTRODUCTION

The Basics

The International Medical Admissions Test (IMAT) is a 100-minute written exam for students who are applying to read medical and veterinary courses at competitive universities across the world.

It is a highly time pressured exam that forces you to apply knowledge in ways you have never thought about before. In this respect simply remembering solutions taught in class or from past papers is not enough.

However, fear not, despite what people say, you can actually prepare for the IMAT! With a little practice you can train your brain to manipulate and apply learnt methodologies to novel problems with ease. The best way to do this is through exposure to as many past/specimen papers as you can.

Preparing for the IMAT

Before going any further, it's important that you understand the optimal way to prepare for the IMAT. Rather than jumping straight into doing mock papers, it's essential that you start by understanding the components and the theory behind the IMAT by using an IMAT textbook. Once you've finished the non-timed practice questions, you can progress to past IMAT papers. These are freely available online at www.uniadmissions.co.uk/IMAT-past-papers and serve as excellent practice. You're strongly advised to use these in combination with the *IMAT Past Paper Worked Solutions* Book so that you can improve your weaknesses. Finally, once you've exhausted past papers, move onto the mock papers in this book.

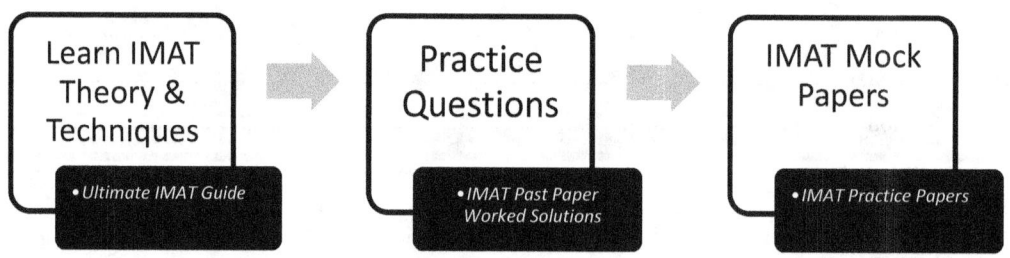

Already seen them all?

So, you've run out of past papers? Well hopefully that is where this book comes in. It contains eight unique mock papers; each compiled by expert IMAT tutors at *UniAdmissions* who scored in the top 10% nationally.

Having successfully gained a place on their course of choice, our tutors are intimately familiar with the IMAT and its associated admission procedures. So, the novel questions presented to you here are of the correct style and difficulty to continue your revision and stretch you to meet the demands of the IMAT.

General Advice

Start Early
It is much easier to prepare if you practice little and often. Start your preparation well in advance; ideally 10 weeks but at the latest within a month. This way you will have plenty of time to complete as many papers as you wish to feel comfortable and won't have to panic and cram just before the test, which is a much less effective and more stressful way to learn. In general, an early start will give you the opportunity to identify the complex issues and work at your own pace.

Prioritise
Some questions in sections can be long and complex – and given the intense time pressure you need to know your limits. It is essential that you don't get stuck with very difficult questions. If a question looks particularly long or complex, mark it for review and move on. You don't want to be caught 5 questions short at the end just because you took more than 3 minutes in answering a challenging multi-step question. If a question is taking too long, choose a sensible answer and move on. Remember that each question carries equal weighting and therefore, you should adjust your timing in accordingly. With practice and discipline, you can get very good at this and learn to maximise your efficiency.

Negative Marking
There is a penalty of -0.4 points for each incorrect answer in the IMAT. This removes the luxury of always being able to guess should you absolutely be not able to figure out the right answer for a question or run behind time. However this does not mean that you should not guess at all. Since each question provides you with 5 possible answers, you have a 20% chance of guessing correctly. Therefore, if you aren't sure (and are running short of time), try to eliminate a couple of answers to increase your chances of getting the question correct. For example, if a question has 5 options and you manage to eliminate 2 options- your chances of getting the question increase from 20% to 33%!

Practice
This is the best way of familiarising yourself with the style of questions and the timing for this section. Although the exam will essentially only test GCSE level knowledge, you are unlikely to be familiar with the style of questions in all sections when you first encounter them. Therefore, you want to be comfortable at using this before you sit the test.

Practising questions will put you at ease and make you more comfortable with the exam. The more comfortable you are, the less you will panic on the test day and the more likely you are to score highly. Initially, work through the questions at your own pace, and spend time carefully reading the questions and looking at any additional data. When it becomes closer to the test, **make sure you practice the questions under exam conditions**.

Past Papers

Official past papers and answers from 2011 onwards are freely available online on our website at www.uniadmissions.co.uk/IMAT-past-papers.

You will undoubtedly get stuck when doing some past paper questions – they are designed to be tricky and the answer schemes don't offer any explanations. Thus, **you're highly advised to acquire a copy of *IMAT Past Paper Worked Solutions*** – a free ebook is available online (see the back of this book for more details).

Repeat Questions

When checking through answers, pay particular attention to questions you have got wrong. If there is a worked answer, look through that carefully until you feel confident that you understand the reasoning, and then repeat the question without help to check that you can do it. If only the answer is given, have another look at the question and try to work out why that answer is correct. This is the best way to learn from your mistakes, and means you are less likely to make similar mistakes when it comes to the test. The same applies for questions which you were unsure of and made an educated guess which was correct, even if you got it right. When working through this book, **make sure you highlight any questions you are unsure of**, this means you know to spend more time looking over them once marked.

No Calculators

You aren't permitted to use calculators in the exam – thus, it is essential that you have strong numerical skills. For instance, you should be able to rapidly convert between percentages, decimals and fractions. You will seldom get questions that would require calculators, but you would be expected to be able to arrive at a sensible estimate. Consider for example:

Estimate 3.962 x 2.322;

3.962 is approximately 4 and 2.323 is approximately 2.33 = 7/3.

Thus, $3.962 \times 2.322 \approx 4 \times \frac{7}{3} = \frac{28}{3} = 9.33$

Since you will rarely be asked to perform difficult calculations, you can use this as a signpost of if you are tackling a question correctly. For example, when solving a physics question, you end up having to divide 8,079 by 357- this should raise alarm bells as calculations in the IMAT are rarely this difficult.

A word on timing...

"If you had all day to do your exam, you would get 100%. But you don't."
Whilst this isn't completely true, it illustrates a very important point. Once you've practiced and know how to answer the questions, the clock is your biggest enemy. This seemingly obvious statement has one very important consequence. **The way to improve your score is to improve your speed.** There is no magic bullet. But there are a great number of techniques that, with practice, will give you significant time gains, allowing you to answer more questions and score more marks.

Timing is tight throughout – **mastering timing is the first key to success**. Some candidates choose to work as quickly as possible to save up time at the end to check back, but this is generally not the best way to do it. Often questions can have a lot of information in them – each time you start answering a question it takes time to get familiar with the instructions and information. By splitting the question into two sessions (the first run-through and the return-to-check) you double the amount of time you spend on familiarising yourself with the data, as you have to do it twice instead of only once. This costs valuable time. In addition, candidates who do check back may spend 2–3 minutes doing so and yet not make any actual changes. Whilst this can be reassuring, it is a false reassurance as it is unlikely to have a significant effect on your actual score. Therefore, it is usually best to pace yourself very steadily, aiming to spend the same amount of time on each question and finish the final question in a section just as time runs out. This reduces the time spent on re-familiarising with questions and maximises the time spent on the first attempt, gaining more marks.

It is essential that you don't get stuck with the hardest questions – no doubt there will be some. In the time spent answering only one of these you may miss out on answering three easier questions. If a question is taking too long, choose a sensible answer and move on. Never see this as giving up or in any way failing, rather it is the smart way to approach a test with a tight time limit. With practice and discipline, you can get very good at this and learn to maximise your efficiency. It is not about being a hero and aiming for full marks – this is almost impossible and very much unnecessary (even Oxbridge will regard any score higher than 7 as exceptional). It is about maximising your efficiency and gaining the maximum possible number of marks within the time you have.

Use the Options:

Some questions may try to overload you with information. When presented with large tables and data, it's essential you look at the answer options so you can focus your mind. This can allow you to reach the correct answer a lot more quickly. Consider the example below:

The table below shows the results of a study investigating antibiotic resistance in staphylococcus populations. A single staphylococcus bacterium is chosen at random from a similar population. Resistance to any one antibiotic is independent of resistance to others.

Calculate the probability that the bacterium selected will be resistant to all four drugs.

A 1 in 10^6
B 1 in 10^{12}
C 1 in 10^{20}
D 1 in 10^{25}
E 1 in 10^{30}
F 1 in 10^{35}

Antibiotic	Number of Bacteria tested	Number of Resistant Bacteria
Benzyl-penicillin	10^{11}	98
Chloramphenicol	10^9	1200
Metronidazole	10^8	256
Erythromycin	10^5	2

Looking at the options first makes it obvious that there is **no need to calculate exact values**- only in powers of 10. This makes your life a lot easier. If you hadn't noticed this, you might have spent well over 90 seconds trying to calculate the exact value when it wasn't even being asked for.

In other cases, you may actually be able to use the options to arrive at the solution quicker than if you had tried to solve the question as you normally would. Consider the example below:

A region is defined by the two inequalities: $x - y^2 > 1 \text{ and } xy > 1$. Which of the following points is in the defined region?

A. (10,3)
B. (10,2)
C. (-10,3)
D. (-10,2)
E. (-10,-3)

Whilst it's possible to solve this question both algebraically or graphically by manipulating the identities, by far **the quickest way is to actually use the options**. Note that options C, D and E violate the second inequality, narrowing down to answer to either A or B. For A: 10 - 3^2 = 1 and thus this point is on the boundary of the defined region and not actually in the region. Thus the answer is B (as 10-4 = 6 > 1.)

In general, it pays dividends to look at the options briefly and see if they can be help you arrive at the question more quickly. Get into this habit early – it may feel unnatural at first but it's guaranteed to save you time in the long run.

Keywords

If you're stuck on a question; pay particular attention to the options that contain key modifiers like "**always**", "**only**", "**all**" as examiners like using them to test if there are any gaps in your knowledge. E.g. the statement "arteries carry oxygenated blood" would normally be true; "All arteries carry oxygenated blood" would be false because the pulmonary artery carries deoxygenated blood.

Manage your Time:

It is highly likely that you will be juggling your revision alongside your normal school studies. Whilst it is tempting to put your A-levels on the back burner falling behind in your school subjects is not a good idea, don't forget that to meet the conditions of your offer should you get one you will need at least one A*. So, time management is key!

Make sure you set aside a dedicated 90 minutes (and much more once you're closer to the exam) to commit to your revision each day. The key here is not to sacrifice too many of your extracurricular activities, everybody needs some down time, but instead to be efficient. Take a look at our list of top tips for increasing revision efficiency below:

1. Create a comfortable work station
2. Declutter and stay tidy
3. Treat yourself to some nice stationery
4. See if music works for you → if not, find somewhere peaceful and quiet to work
5. Turn off your mobile or at least put it into silent mode
6. Silence social media alerts
7. Keep the TV off and out of sight
8. Stay organised with to do lists and revision timetables – more importantly, stick to them!
9. Keep to your set study times and don't bite off more than you can chew
10. Study while you're commuting
11. Adopt a positive mental attitude
12. Get into a routine
13. Consider forming a study group to focus on the harder exam concepts
14. Plan rest and reward days into your timetable – these are excellent incentive for you to stay on track with your study plans!

Keep Fit & Eat Well:

'A car won't work if you fill it with the wrong fuel' - your body is exactly the same. You cannot hope to perform unless you remain fit and well. The best way to do this is not underestimate the importance of healthy eating. Beige, starchy foods will make you sluggish; instead start the day with a hearty breakfast like porridge. Aim for the recommended 'five a day' intake of fruit/veg and stock up on the oily fish or blueberries – the so called "super foods".

When hitting the books, it's essential to keep your brain hydrated. If you get dehydrated you'll find yourself lethargic and possibly developing a headache, neither of which will do any favours for your revision. Invest in a good water bottle that you know the total volume of and keep sipping through the day. Don't forget that the amount of water you should be aiming to drink varies depending on your mass, so calculate your own personal recommended intake as follows: 30 ml per kg per day.

It is well known that exercise boosts your wellbeing and instils a sense of discipline. All of which will reflect well in your revision. It's well worth devoting half an hour a day to some exercise, get your heart rate up, break a sweat, and get those endorphins flowing.

Sleep

It's no secret that when revising you need to keep well rested. Don't be tempted to stay up late revising as sleep actually plays an important part in consolidating long term memory. Instead aim for a minimum of 7 hours good sleep each night, in a dark room without any glow from electronic appliances. Install flux (https://justgetflux.com) on your laptop to prevent your computer from disrupting your circadian rhythm. Aim to go to bed the same time each night and no hitting snooze on the alarm clock in the morning!

IMAT MOCK PAPER | INTRODU

Revision Timetable

Still struggling to get organised? Then try filling in the example revision timetable below, remember to factor in enough time for short breaks, and stick to it! Remember to schedule in several breaks throughout the day and actually use them to do something you enjoy e.g. TV, reading, YouTube etc.

	8AM	10AM	12PM	4PM	6PM	8PM
MONDAY						
TUESDAY						
WEDNESDAY						
THURSDAY						
FRIDAY						
SATURDAY						
SUNDAY						
EXAMPLE DAY	School			Biology	Problem	Physics

low you have a much more accurate idea of the time you're spending on a question. In general, if you've ent >150 seconds on a section 1 question or >90 seconds on a section 2 questions – move on regardless of how close you think you are to solving it.

Getting the most out of Mock Papers

Mock exams can prove invaluable if tackled correctly. Not only do they encourage you to start revision earlier, they also allow you to **practice and perfect your revision technique**. They are often the best way of improving your knowledge base or reinforcing what you have learnt. Probably the best reason for attempting mock papers is to familiarise yourself with the exam conditions of the IMAT as they are particularly tough.

Start Revision Earlier
Thirty five percent of students agree that they procrastinate to a degree that is detrimental to their exam performance. This is partly explained by the fact that they often seem a long way in the future. In the scientific literature this is well recognised, Dr. Piers Steel, an expert on the field of motivation states that *'the further away an event is, the less impact it has on your decisions'*.

Mock exams are therefore a way of giving you a target to work towards and motivate you in the run up to the real thing – every time you do one treat it as the real deal! If you do well then it's a reassuring sign; if you do poorly then it will motivate you to work harder (and earlier!).

Practice and perfect revision techniques
In case you haven't realised already, revision is a skill all to itself, and can take some time to learn. For example, the most common revision techniques including **highlighting and/or re-reading are quite ineffective** ways of committing things to memory. Unless you are thinking critically about something you are much less likely to remember it or indeed understand it.

Mock exams, therefore allow you to test your revision strategies as you go along. Try spacing out your revision sessions so you have time to forget what you have learnt in-between. This may sound counterintuitive but the second time you remember it for longer. Try teaching another student what you have learnt, this forces you to structure the information in a logical way that may aid memory. Always try to question what you have learnt and appraise its validity. Not only does this aid memory but it is also a useful skill for IMAT section 3, Oxbridge interview, and beyond.

Improve your knowledge
The act of applying what you have learnt reinforces that piece of knowledge. A question may ask you to think about a relatively basic concept in a novel way (not cited in textbooks), and so deepen your understanding. Exams rarely test word for word what is in the syllabus, so when running through mock papers try to understand how the basic facts are applied and tested in the exam. As you go through the mocks or past papers take note of your performance and see if you consistently under-perform in specific areas, thus highlighting areas for future study.

Get familiar with exam conditions
Pressure can cause all sorts of trouble for even the most brilliant students. The IMAT is a particularly time pressured exam with high stakes – your future (without exaggerating) does depend on your result to a great extent. The real key to the IMAT is overcoming this pressure and remaining calm to allow you to think efficiently.

Mock exams are therefore an excellent opportunity to devise and perfect your own exam techniques to beat the pressure and meet the demands of the exam. **Don't treat mock exams like practice questions – it's imperative you do them under time conditions.**

Remember! It's better that you make all the mistakes you possibly can now in mock papers and then learn from them so as not to repeat them in the real exam.

Things to have done before using this book

Do the ground work
- Read in detail: the background, methods, and aims of the IMAT as well logistical considerations such as how to take the IMAT in practice. A good place to start is a IMAT textbook like *The Ultimate IMAT Guide* (flick to the back to get a free copy!) which covers all the groundwork but it's also worth looking through the official IMAT site (www.admissionstesting.org/IMAT).
- It is generally a good idea to start re-capping all your GCSE maths and science.
- Practice substituting formulas together to reach a more useful one expressing known variables e.g. $P = IV$ and $V = IR$ can be combined to give $P = V^2/R$ and $P = I^2R$. Remember that calculators are not permitted in the exam, so get comfortable doing more complex long addition, multiplication, division, and subtraction.
- Get comfortable rapidly converting between percentages, decimals, and fractions.
- Practice developing logical arguments and structuring essays with an obvious introduction, main body, and ending.
- These are all things which are easiest to do alongside your revision for exams before the summer break. Not only gaining a head start on your IMAT revision but also complimenting your year 12 studies well.
- Discuss scientific problems with others - propose experiments and state what you think the result would be. Be ready to defend your argument. This will rapidly build your scientific understanding for section 2 but also prepare you well for an oxbridge interview.
- Read through the IMAT syllabus before you start tackling whole papers. This is absolutely essential. It contains several stated formulae, constants, and facts that you are expected to apply - or may just be an answer in their own right. Familiarising yourself with the syllabus is also a quick way of teaching yourself the additional information other exam boards may learn which you do not. Sifting through the whole IMAT syllabus is a time-consuming process so we have done it for you. **Be sure to flick through the syllabus checklist** later on, which also doubles up as a great revision aid for the night before!

Ease in gently
With the ground work laid, there's still no point in adopting exam conditions straight away. Instead invest in a beginner's guide to the IMAT, which will not only describe in detail the background and theory of the exam, but take you through section by section what is expected. *The Ultimate IMAT Guide: 800 Practice Questions* is the most popular IMAT textbook – you can get a free copy by flicking to the back of this book.

When you are ready to move on to past papers, take your time and puzzle your way through all the questions. Really try to understand solutions. A past paper question won't be repeated in your real exam, so don't rote learn methods or facts. Instead, focus on applying prior knowledge to formulate your own approach.

If you're really struggling and have to take a sneak peek at the answers, then practice thinking of alternative solutions, or arguments for essays. It is unlikely that your answer will be more elegant or succinct than the model answer, but it is still a good task for encouraging creativity with your thinking. Get used to thinking outside the box!

Accelerate and Intensify

Start adopting exam conditions after you've done two past papers. Don't forget that **it's the time pressure that makes the IMAT hard** – if you had as long as you wanted to sit the exam you would probably get 100%. If you're struggling to find comprehensive answers to past papers then *IMAT Past Papers Worked Solutions* contains detailed explained answers to every IMAT past paper question and essay (flick to the back to get a free copy).

Doing all the past papers from 2009 – present is a good target for your revision. Note that the IMAT syllabus changed in 2009 so questions before this date may no longer be relevant. In any case, choose a paper and proceed with strict exam conditions. Take a short break and then mark your answers before reviewing your progress. For revision purposes, as you go along, keep track of those questions that you guess – these are equally as important to review as those you get wrong.

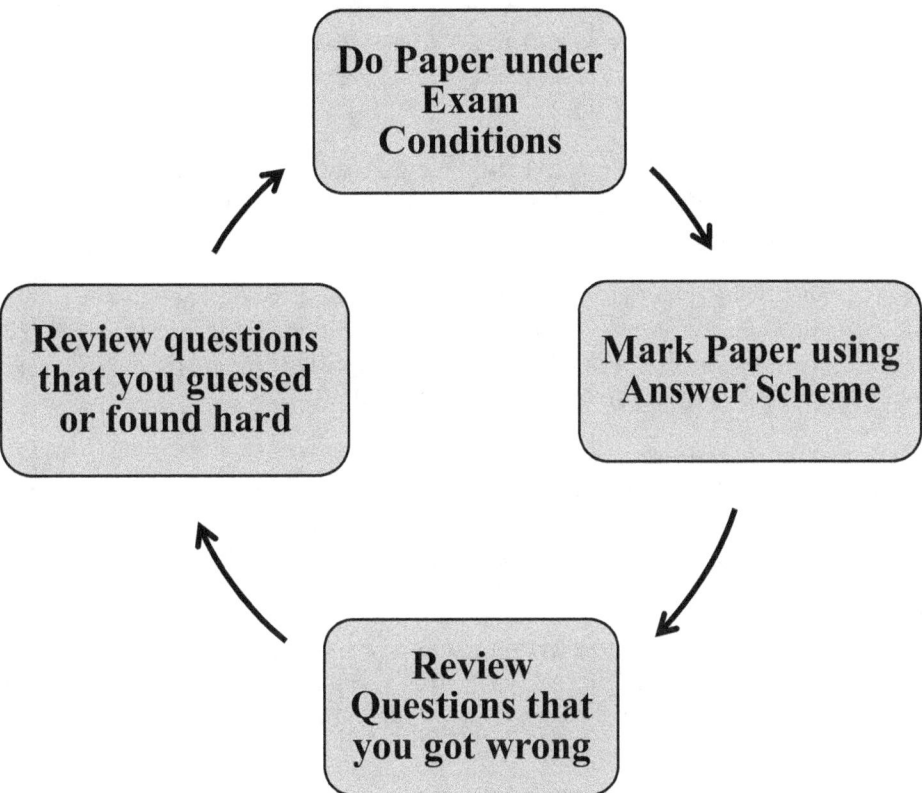

Once you've exhausted all the past papers, move on to tackling the unique mock papers in this book. In general, you should aim to complete one to two mock papers every night in the ten days preceding your exam.

Section 1: An Overview

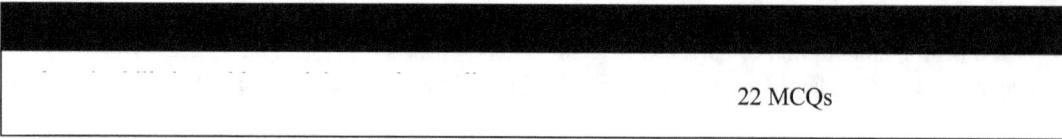

22 MCQs

This is the first section of the IMAT, comprising what most people describe as the classic IQ test style questions. Giving you one hour to answer 35 questions testing your ability to think critically, solve problems, and handle data. Breaking things down you realise that you are left with approximately 100 seconds per question. Remember though that this not only includes reasoning your answers, but also reading passages of text and/or analysing diagrams or graphs.

Not all the questions are of equal difficulty and so as you work through the past material it is certainly worth learning to recognise quickly which questions you need to skip to avoid getting bogged down. If it comes to it and you do not have enough time to go back to any skipped questions at the end, you always have a 20% chance of getting the answer correct with a guess!

Critical thinking questions
These types of question will generally present you with a passage of text or a methodology for an experiment and ask you to do one of three things: identify a conclusion, identify and assumption or flaw, or give an argument to either strengthen or weaken the statement.

The ability to filter through irrelevant material is essential with these questions as well as a solid grasp of the English language. Remember to only use the information given to you in your reasoning and never be too general with your conclusions – seek direct evidence in the information given. Critical thinking questions are definitely an example of when it is **best to read the question first**!

Problem solving questions
The problems in section 1 are often very wordy and complex, therefore it is often useful to turn the prose of the question into a series of equations. For example, being able to turn the sentence "Megan is half as tall as Elin" into "2M = E" should become second nature to you. Trial and error is not a method you should adopt for any questions in section 1 as it is far too time consuming.

As you are working through the preparation material try to get used to recognising which questions can be aided by drawing a quick diagram. This could apply to questions asking about timetables, orders, sequences, or spatial relationships. Remember it doesn't have to be pretty, merely help you organise your thoughts!

Data handling questions
These questions will undoubtedly require you to work with numbers, often calculating percentages or frequencies. Again, reading the question first can help you save time here, directing your attention to the relevant information in the passage. When analysing tables or graphs always check the following:

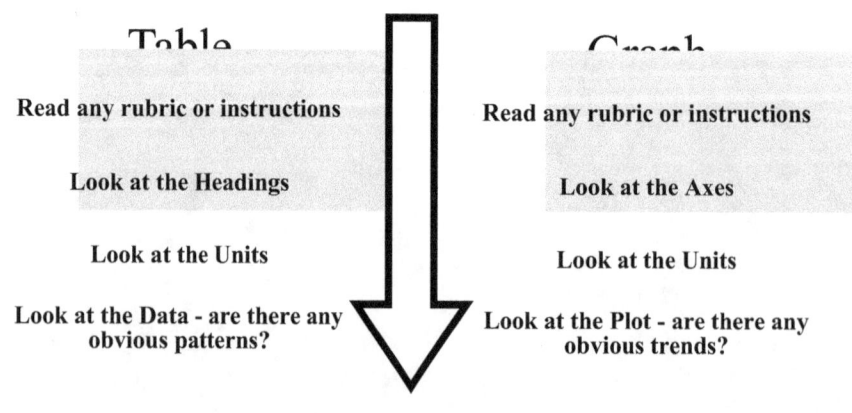

Sections 2, 3 & 4: An Overview

What will you be tested on?	No. of Questions	Duration
Ability to recall, understand and apply scientific knowledge and principles of biology, chemistry, physics, and maths. Usually the sections that students find the hardest.	38 MCQs	65 Minutes

If you're short of time, then these sections are where to focus. Undoubtedly the most time pressured section of the IMAT (requiring you to answer a question every 100 seconds) but also the section where candidates improve the fastest. These sections draw on your knowledge of biology, chemistry, physics, and maths.

Biology
Generally, the biology questions require the least amount of time and are often where you can rely on making up lost time from harder questions. Most of biology questions rely on you being able to recall facts rather than interpret data or solve equations, so some good old-fashioned text book revision will prepare you well for these questions.

Chemistry
If you're taking the IMAT you will undoubtedly be studying chemistry at A-level as it is a requirement of all medical schools. Conceptually therefore, you should be in the clear, however, balancing complex equations or processing lengthy calculations can be time consuming.

Practicing with mock papers is essentially in combating this – really focus on extracting what the question is asking for as quickly as possible. In addition to the equations on the subsequent pages you must be comfortable with converting between litres, dm^3, cm^3, and mm^3 as well as using Avogadro's constant in calculations.

Physics
Physics is by far the most common subject that students drop moving on to AS-level, meaning these questions are the most poorly answered. There is a large variation in physics specifications between GCSE exam boards, so **before you do anything else read through the IMAT syllabus and commit all the stated equations and constants to memory** (helpfully highlighted in bold type on the revision checklist).

Physics questions will almost always require a two-step solution, normally forcing you to combine and re-arrange equations. All answers must be given in SI units which actually benefits you, by looking at the units you can often derive the equation – for example speed in m/s is calculated as distance(m) / time(s). It is also worth becoming fluent with the terminology for orders of magnitude in measurements (see right).

Maths
Maths is the single most important component of section 2, a question topic in its own right but also applied in chemistry, physics, and section 1. Just remember to limit yourself to GCSE knowledge in the maths questions and don't overcomplicate things. As a bare minimum for preparation you should practice applying the quadratic formula, completing the square, and finding the difference between 2 squares.

Factor	Text	Symbol
10^{12}	Tera	T
10^{9}	Giga	G
10^{6}	Mega	M
10^{3}	Kilo	k
10^{2}	Hecto	h
10^{-1}	Deci	d
10^{-2}	Centi	c
10^{-3}	Milli	m
10^{-6}	Micro	μ
10^{-9}	Nano	n
10^{-12}	Pico	p

How to use this Book

If you have done everything this book has described so far then you should be well equipped to meet the demands of the IMAT, and therefore **the mock papers in the rest of this book should ONLY be completed under exam conditions**.

This means:

- Absolute silence – no TV or music
- Absolute focus – no distractions such as eating your dinner
- Strict time constraints – no pausing half way through
- No checking the answers as you go
- Give yourself a maximum of three minutes between sections – keep the pressure up
- Complete the entire paper before marking
- Mark harshly

In practice this means setting aside two hours in an evening to find a quiet spot without interruptions and tackle the paper. Completing one mock paper every evening in the week running up to the exam would be an ideal target.

- Tackle the paper as you would in the exam.
- Return to mark your answers, but mark harshly if there's any ambiguity.
- Highlight any areas of concern.
- If warranted read up on the areas you felt you underperformed to reinforce your knowledge.
- If you inadvertently learnt anything new by muddling through a question, go and tell somebody about it to reinforce what you've discovered.

Finally relax... the IMAT is an exhausting exam, concentrating so hard continually for two hours will take its toll. So, being able to relax and switch off is essential to keep yourself sharp for exam day! Make sure you reward yourself after you finish marking your exam.

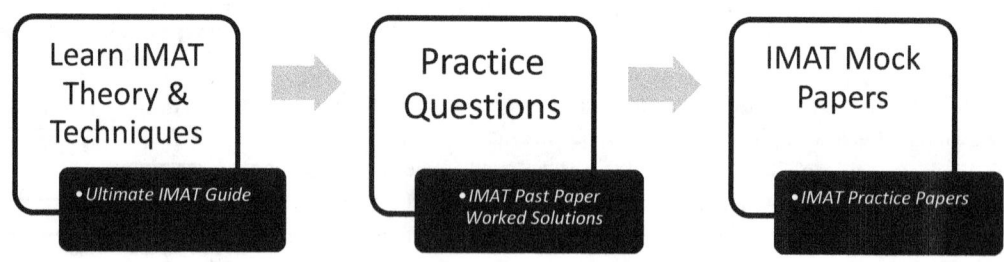

Scoring Tables

Use these to keep a record of your scores from past papers – you can then easily see which paper you should attempt next (always the one with the lowest score).

SECTION 1	1st Attempt	2nd Attempt	3rd Attempt
2011			
2012			
2013			
2014			
2015			
2016			
2017			
2018			

SECTION 2	1st Attempt	2nd Attempt	3rd Attempt
2011			
2012			
2013			
2014			
2015			
2016			
2017			
2018			

SECTION 3	1st Attempt	2nd Attempt	3rd Attempt
2011			
2012			
2013			
2014			
2015			
2016			
2017			
2018			

SECTION 4	1st Attempt	2nd Attempt	3rd Attempt
2011			
2012			
2013			
2014			
2015			
2016			
2017			
2018			

And the same again here but with our mocks instead.

SECTION 1	1st Attempt	2nd Attempt	3rd Attempt
Mock A			
Mock B			
Mock C			
Mock D			

SECTION 2	1st Attempt	2nd Attempt	3rd Attempt
Mock A			
Mock B			
Mock C			
Mock D			

SECTION 3	1st Attempt	2nd Attempt	3rd Attempt
Mock A			
Mock B			
Mock C			
Mock D			

SECTION 4	1st Attempt	2nd Attempt	3rd Attempt
Mock A			
Mock B			
Mock C			
Mock D			

MOCK PAPER A

Section 1

Question 1:
The Dolomite mountain range, which borders the Alps, is located in which country?

A) Italy B) France C) Germany D) Denmark E) Spain

Question 2:
The Marriage of Figaro is an opera written by which 18th century composer?

A) Beethoven
B) Mozart
C) Tchaikovsky
D) Chopin
E) Rimsky-Korsakov

Question 3:
Which Ancient empire built the city of Tenochtitlan in modern day Mexico?

A) Aztec B) Inca C) Babylon D) Rome E) Maya

Question 4:
Which Dutch artists painted *Girl with a Pearl Earring*?

A) Vincent Van Gogh
B) Johannes Vermeer
C) Sandro Boticelli
D) Pablo Picasso
E) Rembrandt

Question 5:
The speech which begins 'Friends, Romans, Countrymen, lend me your ears' is from which play by Shakespeare?

A) Othello B) Romeo & Juliet C) Anthony & Cleopatra D) The Merchant of Venice E) Julius Caesar

Question 6:
What ruler was crowned emperor of the Holy Roman Empire on Christmas Day of 800 AD?

A) Robert the Bruce B) Edward I C) Charlemagne D) Julius Caesar E) Charles the Bald

Question 7:
The Harlem Renaissance was a 20th Century artistic and poetic movement based in which city?

A) Paris
B) Madrid
C) New York
D) San Francisco
E) Chicago

Question 8:
The Knights Hospitalier formerly governed which EU member state?

A) Italy
B) Malta
C) Spain
D) France
E) Cyprus

Question 9:
Which British prime minister left office after nearly 12 years in power in 1990?

A) John Major
B) Gordon Brown
C) Tony Blair
D) Harold Wilson
E) Margaret Thatcher

Question 10:
Io and Europa are both moons of which planet?

A) Jupiter   B) Saturn   C) Uranus   D) Neptune   E) Pluto

Question 11:
In 2016 the Colombian government signed a peace accord with members of which militant group?

A) FARC   C) Al-Qaida   D) Shining Path   E) ETA
B) IRA

Question 12:
The Metamorphoses is a work of Latin poetry by which author?
A) Homer   D) Ovid
B) Dante   E) Plato
C) Virgil

Question 13:
Car A has a fuel tank capacity of 30 gallons and achieves 40mpg. Car B on the other hand has a fuel tank capacity of 50 gallons but only achieves 30mpg. Both cars drive until they run out of fuel. If car A starts with a full tank of petrol and travels 200 miles further than car B, how full was car B's fuel tank?

F) 1/5   G) 1/4   H) 1/3   I) 1/2   J) 2/3

Question 14:
The keypad to a safe comprises the digits 1 - 9. The code itself can be of indeterminate length. The code is therefore set by choosing a reference number so that when a code is entered the average of all the numbers entered must equal the chosen reference number.

Which of the following is true?

A) If the reference number was set greater than 9, the safe would be locked forever.
B) This safe is extremely insecure as if random digits were pressed for long enough it would average out at the correct reference number.
C) More than one number is always required to achieve the reference number.
D) All of the above are true.
E) None of the above are true.

Question 15:
The use of antibiotics is one of the major paradoxes in modern medicine. Antibiotics themselves provide a selection pressure to drive the evolution of antibiotic resistant strains of bacteria. This is largely due to the rapid growth rate of bacterial colonies and asexual cell division. As such a widespread initiative is in place to limit the prescription of antibiotics.
Which of the following is a fair assumption?

A) Antibiotic resistance is impossible to avoid as it is driven by evolution.
B) If bacteria reproduced at a slower rate antibiotic resistance would not be such an issue.
C) Medicine always creates more problems than it solves.
D) In the past antibiotics were used frivolously.
E) All of the above could be possible.

The information below relates to questions 16 – 20:

The Spaghetti Bolognese recipe below serves 10 people and each portion contains 300 kcal.
- 1kg mince
- 220g pancetta, diced
- 30g crushed garlic
- 1kg tinned tomatoes
- 300g diced onions
- 300g sliced mushrooms
- 200g grated cheese

Question 16:
What quantity of cheese is required to prepare a meal for 350 people?

A) 0.7kg   B) 7kg   C) 70kg   D) 700kg   E) 7000kg

Question 17:
If 12 portions represent 120% of an individual's recommended calorific intake, what is that individuals recommended calorific intake?

A) 2600kcal   B) 2800kcal   C) 3000kcal   D) 3200kcal   E) 3400kcal

Question 18:
The recommended ratio of pasta to Bolognese is 4:1. If cooking for 30 people how much pasta should be used?

A) 30.3kg   B) 36.6kg   C) 42.9kg   D) 49.2kg   E) 55.5kg

Question 19:
What is the ratio of onions to the rest of the ingredients if garlic and pancetta are ignored?

F) 1/2.05   G) 1/3.9   H) 1/6.7   I) 1/9.3   J) 1/10

Question 20:
It takes 4 minutes to prepare the ingredients per portion, and a further 8 minutes per portion to cook. Simon has ample preparation space but is limited to cooking 8 portions at a time. What is the shortest period of time it would take him to turn all the ingredients into a meal for 25 people, assuming he didn't start cooking until all the ingredients were prepared?

A) 3 hours
B) 3 hours 40
C) 4 hours
D) 4 hours 40
E) 5 hours

Question 21:
A square sheet of paper is 20cms long. How many times must it be folded in half before it covers an area of 12.5cm^2?

A) 3   B) 4   C) 5   D) 6   E) 7

Question 22:
50% of an isolated population contract a new strain of resistant Malaria. Only 20% are symptomatic of which 10% are female. What percentage of the total population do symptomatic males represent?

A) 1%
B) 9%
C) 80%
D) 15%
E) 10%

END OF SECTION

Section 2

Question 23:
Which of the following cannot be classified as an organ?
1. Blood
2. Bone
3. Larynx
4. Pituitary Gland
5. Prostate
6. Skeletal Muscle
7. Skin

A) 1 and 6   B) 2 and 3   C) 5 and 7   D) 1 and 5   E) 1, 4, 5 and 6

Question 24:
An increase in aerobic respiratory rate could be associated with which of the following physiological changes?
1. A larger percentage of water vapour in expired air
2. Increased expired CO_2
3. Increased inspired O_2
4. Perspiration
5. Vasodilatation

A) 3 only
B) 1 and 2 only
C) 1, 2 and 3 only
D) 2, 3 and 5
E) All of the above

Question 25:
The nephron is to the kidney, as the _____ is to striated muscle:

A) Actin filament
B) Artery
C) Myofibril
D) Sarcomere
E) Vein

Question 26:
A diabetic patient's glucagon and insulin levels are measured over 4 hours. During this time the patient is given two large boluses of glucose. A graphical representation of this is shown below.

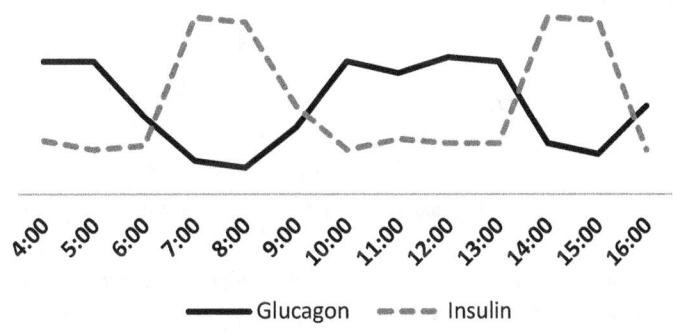

At which times would you expect the patients' blood glucose to be greatest?

A) 05:00 and 12:00
B) 07:00 and 14:00
C) 08:00 and 15:00
D) 10:00 and 13:00
E) 06:00, 10:00 and 16:00

Question 27:
In addition to the A, B or O classification, blood groups can also be distinguished by the presence of Rhesus antigen (Rh). Care must be taken in blood transfusion as once blood types are mixed a Rh -ve individual will mount an immune response against Rh +ve blood. This is particular well exemplified in haemolytic disease of the newborn – where a Rh-ve mother carries a Rh+ve foetus.

Applying what is written here and your knowledge of the human immune system, explain why the mother's first child would be relatively safe and unaffected, yet further offspring would be at high risk.

A) The first pregnancy is always such a shock to the body it compromises the immune system.
B) Antibodies take longer than 9 months to produce and mature to an active state.
C) First born children are immunologically privileged.
D) There is a high risk of haemorrhage to both mother and child during birth.
E) Plasma T cells require time to multiply to lethal levels.

Question 28:
At present a large effort is being made to produce tailored patient care. One of the ultimate goals of this is to be able to grow personal, genetically identical organs for those with end stage organ failure. This process will first require the harbouring of what cell type?

A) Cells from the organ that is failing
B) Haematopoietic stem cells
C) Embryonic stem cells
D) Adult stem cells
E) All of the above

Question 29:
In relation to the human genome, which of the following are correct?

1. The DNA genome is coded by 4 different bases.
2. The sugar backbone of the DNA strand is formed of glucose.
3. DNA is found in the nucleus of bacteria.

A) 1 only
B) 2 only
C) 3 only
D) 1 and 2
E) 1 and 3
F) 2 and 3
G) 1, 2 and 3

Question 30:
Animal cells contain organelles that take part in vital processes. Which of the following is true?

1. The majority of energy production by animal cells occurs in the mitochondria.
2. The cell wall protects the animal cell membrane from outside pressure differences.
3. The endoplasmic reticulum plays a role in protein synthesis.

A) 1 only
B) 2 only
C) 3 only
D) 1 and 2
E) 2 and 3
F) 1 and 3
G) 1, 2 and 3

Question 31:
With regards to animal mitochondria, which of the following is correct?

A) Mitochondria are not necessary for aerobic respiration.
B) Mitochondria are the sole cause of sperm cell movement.
C) The majority of DNA replication happens inside mitochondria.
D) Mitochondria are more abundant in fat cells than in skeletal muscle.
E) The majority of protein synthesis occurs in mitochondria.
F) Mitochondria are enveloped by a double membrane.

Question 32:
In relation to bacteria, which of the following is **FALSE**?

A) Bacteria always lead to disease.
B) Bacteria contain plasmid DNA.
C) Bacteria do not contain mitochondria.
D) Bacteria have a cell wall and a plasma membrane.
E) Some bacteria are susceptible to antibiotics.

Question 33:
In relation to bacterial replication, which of the following is correct?

A) Bacteria undergo sexual reproduction.
B) Bacteria have a nucleus.
C) Bacteria carry genetic information on circular plasmids.
D) Bacterial genomes are formed of RNA instead of DNA.
E) Bacteria require gametes to replicate.

Question 34:
Which of the following are correct regarding active transport?

A) ATP is necessary and sufficient for active transport.
B) ATP is not necessary but sufficient for active transport.
C) The relative concentrations of the material being transported have little impact on the rate of active transport.
D) Transport proteins are necessary and sufficient for active transport.
E) Active transport relies on transport proteins that are powered by an electrochemical gradient.

Question 35:
Concerning mammalian reproduction, which of the following is **FALSE**?

A) Fertilisation involves the fusion of two gametes.
B) Reproduction is sexual and the offspring display genetic variation.
C) Reproduction relies upon the exchange of genetic material.
D) Mammalian gametes are diploid cells produced via meiosis.
E) Embryonic growth requires carefully controlled mitosis.

MOCK PAPER A — SECTION TWO

Question 36:
Which of the following apply to Mendelian inheritance?

1. It only applies to plants.
2. It treats different traits as either dominant or recessive.
3. Heterozygotes have a 25% chance of expressing a recessive trait.

A) 1 only   C) 3 only   E) 1 and 3   G) All of the above
B) 2 only   D) 1 and 2   F) 2 and 3

Question 37:
Which of the following statements are correct?

A) Hormones are secreted into the blood stream and act over long distances at specific target organs.
B) Hormones are substances that almost always cause muscles to contract.
C) Hormones have no impact on the nervous or enteric systems.
D) Hormones are always derived from food and never synthesised.
E) Hormones act rapidly to restore homeostasis.

Question 38:
With regard to neuronal signalling in the body, which of the following are true?

1. Neuronal transmission can be caused by both electrical and chemical stimulation.
2. Synapses ultimately result in the production of an electrical current for signal transduction.
3. All synapses in humans are electrical and unidirectional.

A) 1 only   C) 3 only   E) 1 and 3   G) 1, 2 and 3
B) 2 only   D) 1 and 2   F) 2 and 3

Question 39:
What is the **primary** reason that pH is controlled so tightly in humans?

A) To allow rapid protein synthesis.
B) To allow for effective digestion throughout the GI tract.
C) To ensure ions can function properly in neural signalling.
D) To prevent changes in electrical charge in polypeptide chains.
E) To prevent changes in core body temperature.

Question 40:
Which of the following statements are correct regarding bacterial cell walls?

1. It confers bacteria protection against external environmental stimuli.
2. It is an evolutionary remnant and now has little functional significance in most bacteria.
3. It is made up primarily of glucose in bacteria.

A) Only 1   D) 1 and 2   G) 1, 2 and 3
B) Only 2   E) 2 and 3
C) Only 3   F) 1 and 3

END OF SECTION

Section 3

Question 41:
The pH of a solution has the greatest effect on which type of interaction?

A) Van der Waals
B) Induced dipole
C) Ionic bonding
D) Metallic interaction
E) Hydrogen bonding

Question 42:
When comparing different isotopes of the same element, which of the following may change?
1. Atomic number
2. Mass number
3. Number of electrons
4. Chemical reactivity

A) 1 only
B) 1 and 2 only
C) 3 only
D) 2 and 3 only
E) All of the above

Question 43:
From which of the following elemental groups are you most likely to find a catalyst?

A) Alkali Metals
B) d-block elements
C) Alkaline Earth Metals
D) Noble Gases
E) Halogens

Question 44:
1.338kg of francium are mixed in a reaction vessel with an excess of distilled water. What volume will the hydrogen produced occupy at room temperature and pressure?

A) $20.4dm^3$
B) $36dm^3$
C) $40.8dm^3$
D) $60.12dm^3$
E) $72dm^3$

Question 45:
The composition of a compound is Carbon 30%, Hydrogen 40%, Fluorine 20%, and Chlorine 10%.
What is the empirical formula of this compound?

A) CH_2FCl
B) $C_3H_2F_2Cl$
C) C_3H_4FCl
D) $C_3H_4F_2Cl$
E) $C_4H_4F_2Cl$

Question 46:
What is the actual molecular formula of the compound in question 13 if the M_r is 340.5?

A) $C_3H_4F_2Cl$
B) $C_6H_8F_4Cl_2$
C) $C_9H_{12}F_6Cl_3$
D) $C_{12}H_{16}F_8Cl_4$
E) $C_{15}H_{20}F_{10}Cl_5$

Question 47:
1.2×10^{10} kg of sugar is dissolved in 4×10^{12} L of distilled water. What is the concentration?

A) 3×10^{-2} g/dL
B) 3×10^{-1} g/dL
C) 3×10^1 g/dL
D) 3×10^2 g/dL
E) 3×10^3 g/dL

Question 48:
Which of the following is not essential for the progression of an exothermic chemical reaction?

A) Presence of a catalyst
B) Increase in entropy
C) Achieving activation energy
D) Attaining an electron configuration more closely resembling that of a noble gas
E) None of the above

Question 49:
What is a common use of cationic surfactants?

A) Shampoo
B) Lubricant
C) Cosmetics
D) Detergents
E) All of the above

Question 50:
Which of the following most accurately defines an isotope?

A) An isotope is an atom of an element that has the same number of protons in the nucleus but a different number of neutrons orbiting the nucleus.
B) An isotope is an atom of an element that has the same number of neutrons in the nucleus but a different number of protons orbiting the nucleus.
C) An isotope is any atom of an element that can be split to produce nuclear energy.
D) An isotope is an atom of an element that has the same number of protons in the nucleus but a different number of neutrons in the nucleus.
E) An isotope is an atom of an element that has the same number of protons in the nucleus but a different number of electrons orbiting it.

Question 51:
Which of the following is an example of a displacement reaction?

1. $Fe + SnSO_4 \rightarrow FeSO_4 + Sn$
2. $Cl_2 + 2KBr \rightarrow Br_2 + 2KCl$
3. $H_2SO_4 + Mg \rightarrow MgSO_4 + H_2$
4. $NaHCO_3 + HCl \rightarrow NaCl + CO_2 + H_2O$

A) 1 only
B) 1 and 2 only
C) 2 and 3 only
D) 3 and 4 only
E) 1, 2 and 3 only
F) 1, 2, 3 and 4

Question 52:
What values of **a**, **b** and **c** are needed to balance the equation below?

$aCa(OH)_2 + bH_3PO_4 \rightarrow Ca_3(PO_4)_2 + cH_2O$

A) a = 3 b = 2 c = 6
B) a = 2 b = 2 c = 4
C) a = 3 b = 2 c = 1
D) a = 1 b = 2 c = 3
E) a = 4 b = 2 c = 6
F) a = 3 b = 2 c = 4

END OF SECTION

Section 4

Question 53:
A crocodile's tail weighs 30kg. Its head weighs as much as the tail and one half of the body and legs. The body and legs together weigh as much as the tail and head combined.

What is the total weight of the crocodile?

A) 220kg   B) 240kg   C) 260kg   D) 280kg   E) 300kg

Question 54:
A body is travelling at x ms^{-1} with y J of kinetic energy. After a period of retardation the kinetic energy of the body is $1/16y$. Assuming that the mass of the body has remained constant what is its new velocity?

A) $1/196x$ B) $1/16x$ C) $1/8x$ D) $1/4x$ E) $4x$

Question 55:
Which of the following is a unit equivalent to the Volt?

A) $A.\Omega^{-1}$ B) $J.C^{-1}$ C) $W.s^{-1}$ D) $C.s$ E) $W.C.\Omega$

Question 56:
Complete the sentence below:
A voltmeter is connected in _____ and therefore has _____ resistance; whereas an ammeter is connected in _____ and has _____ resistance.

A) Parallel, zero, parallel, infinite
B) Parallel, zero, series, infinite
C) Parallel, infinite, series, zero
D) Series, zero, parallel, infinite
E) Series, infinite, parallel, zero

Question 57:
A body "A" of mass 12kg travelling at 15m/s undergoes inelastic collision with a fixed, stationary object "B" of mass 20kg over a period of 0.5 seconds. After the collision body A has a new velocity of 3m/s. What force must have been dissipated during the collision?

A) 288N   B) 298N   C) 308N   D) 318N   E) 328N

Question 58:
What process is illustrated here: $^{14}_{6}C \rightarrow {}^{14}_{7}N + x$

A) Thermal decomposition   C) Beta decay
B) Alpha decay   D) Gamma decay

Question 59:
A radio dish is broadcasting messages into deep space on a 20 Hz radio frequency of wavelength 3km. With every hour how much further does the signal travel into deep space?

A) 200,000 km   C) 232,000 km   E) 264,000 km
B) 216,000 km   D) 248,000 km

Question 60:

A formula: $\sqrt[3]{\frac{z(x+y)(l+m-n)}{3}}$ is given. Would you expect this formula to calculate:

A) A length
B) An area
C) A volume
D) A volume of rotation
E) A geometric average

END OF PAPER

MOCK PAPER B

Section 1

Question 1:
In 2016, the satellite *Juno* entered ordbit around which planet?

A) Neptune
B) Uranus
C) Mars
D) Saturn
E) Jupiter

Question 2:
Which of these rivers is NOT located in Europe?

A) Danube B) Seine C) Rhine D) Elbe E) Yellow

Question 3:
The American Declaration of Independence was signed on the 4th of July of what year?

A) 1815
B) 1789
C) 1688
D) 1776
E) 1492

Question 4:
Which major figure of 20th Century politics was released from prison in 1990?

A) Martin Luther King
B) Malcolm X
C) Nelson Mandela
D) Robert Mugabe
E) General Nasser

Question 5:

The international agreement to reduce greenhouse gas emissions agreed by 192 countries in 1997 was signed in what city?

A) New York
B) Tokyo
C) Seoul
D) Kyoto
E) Paris

Question 6:
Marie Curie died as a result of her research into what?

A) Poisons B) Acids C) Fire D) Radiation E) Monkeys

Question 7:
Who famously said "I disapprove of what you say, but I will defend to the death your right to say it"?

A) Rene Descartes
B) Roger Bacon
C) Voltaire
D) Baruch Spinoza
E) Desideridus Erasmus

Question 8:
Which of these countries was never part of the United Republic of Yugoslavia?

A) Bosnia
B) Serbia
C) Macedonia
D) Hungary
E) Slovenia

Question 9:
Which of these is not a novel by Jane Austen?

A) Sense & Sensibility
B) Pride & Prejudice
C) Emma
D) Mansfield Park
E) Clarissa

Question 10:
Bastille Day is celebrated every year in France on what day?

A) 4th of July
B) 5th of November
C) 8th of August
D) 14th of July
E) 1st of December

Question 11:
The phrase "Hell is other people" is associated with which French philosopher?

A) Jean-Paul Sartre
B) Albert Camus
C) Freidrich Nietzsche
D) Jean-Jacques Rousseau
E) Rene Descartes

Question 12:
Siddharta Gautama is the real historical name of which religious figure?

A) Jesus Christ
B) Zoroaster
C) Buddha
D) Moses
E) Guru Nanak

The information below relates to questions 13 – 17:

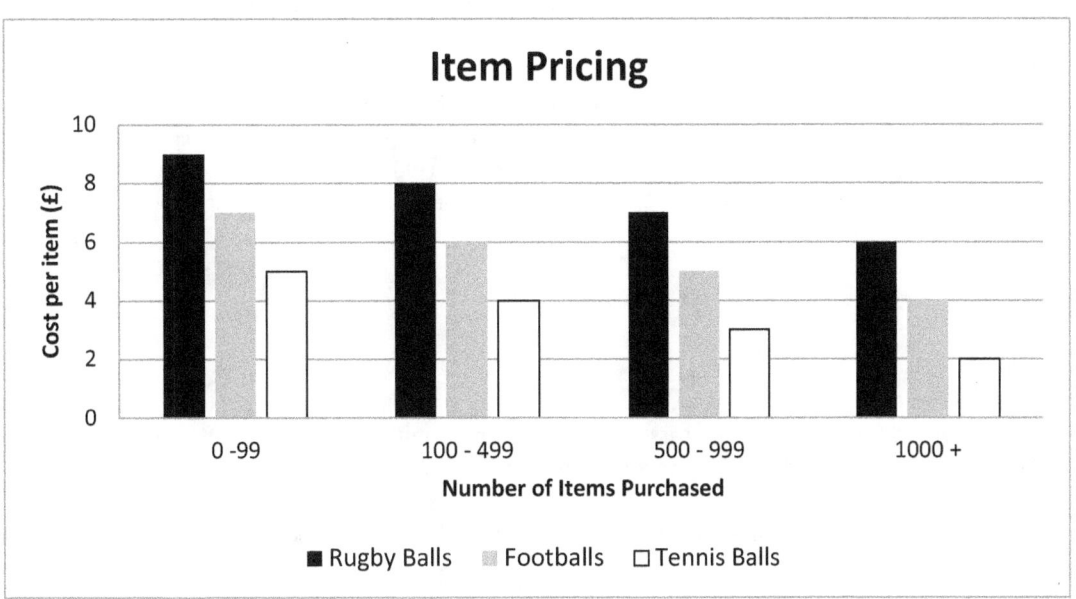

The graph above shows item pricing from a wholesaler. The wholesaler is happy to deliver for a cost of £35 to companies or £5 to individuals. Any order over the cost of £100 qualifies for free delivery. Items are defined as how they come to the wholesaler therefore 1 item = 2 rugby balls or 1 football or 5 tennis balls.

Question 13:
What is the total cost to an individual purchasing 12 rugby balls and 120 tennis balls?

A) £174 B) £179 C) £208 D) £534 E) £588

Question 14:
A private gym wishes to purchase 10 of everything, how short are they of the free delivery boundary?

A) £5.00
B) £5.01
C) £10.00
D) £10.01
E) They are already over the minimum

Question 15:
What is the most number of balls that can be bought by an individual with £1,000 pounds.

A) 200 B) 250 C) 500 D) 1,000 E) 1,250

Question 16:
The wholesaler sells all his products for a profit of 120%. If he sells £1,320 worth of goods at his prices, what did he spend on acquiring them himself?

A) £400 B) £600 C) £800 D) £1,100 E) £1,120

Question 17:
If the wholesaler pays 25% tax on the amount over £12,000 pounds; how much tax does he pay when receiving an order of 2,000 of each item?

A) £2,000 B) £3,000 C) £4,000 D) £5,000 E) £6,000

Question 18:
There are four houses on a street. Lucy, Vicky, and Shannon live in adjacent houses. Shannon has a black dog named Chrissie, Lucy has a white Persian cat and Vicky has a red parrot that shouts obscenities. The owner of a four-legged pet has a blue door. Vicky has a neighbour with a red door. Either a cat or bird owner has a white door. Lucy lives opposite a green door. Vicky and Shannon are not neighbours. What colour is Lucy's door?

A) Green
B) Red
C) White
D) Blue
E) Cannot tell

Question 19:
A train driver runs a service between Cardiff and Merthyr. On average a one-way trip takes 40 minutes to drive but he requires 5 minutes to unload passengers and a further 5 minutes to pick up new ones. As the crow flies the distance between Cardiff and Merthyr is 22 miles.

Assuming he works an 8-hour shift with two 20-minute breaks, and when he arrives to work the first train is already loaded with passengers how far does he travel?

A) 132 B) 143 C) 154 D) 176 E) 198

Question 20:
The massive volume of traffic that travels down the M4 corridor regularly leads to congestion at times of commute morning and evening. A case is being made by local councils in congestion areas to introduce relief lanes thus widening the motorway in an attempt to relieve the congestion. This would involve introducing either a new 2 or 4 lanes to the motorway on average costing 1 million pound per lane per 10 miles.

Many conservationist groups are concerned as this will involve the destruction of large areas of countryside either side of the motorway. They argue that the side of a motorway is a unique habitat with many rare species residing there.

The local councils argue that with many hundreds if not thousands of cars siding idle on the motorway pumping pollutants out into the surrounding areas, it is better for the wildlife if the congestion is eased and traffic can flow through. The councils have also remarked that if congestion is eased there would be less money needed to repair the roads from car incidents with could in theory be given to the conservationist groups as a grant.

Which of the following is assumed in this passage?

A) Wildlife living on the side of the motorway cannot be re-homed.
B) Congestion causes car incidents.
C) Relief lanes have been proven to improve traffic jams.
D) A and B.
E) B and C.
F) All of the above.
G) None of the above.

Question 21:
In 4 years time I will be one third the age that my brother will be next year. In 20 years time he will be double my age. How old am I?

A) 4
B) 9
C) 15
D) 17
E) 23

Question 22:
A television is delivered in a box that has volume 60% larger than that of the television. The television is 150cm x 100cm x 10m. How much surplus volume is there?

A) $0.09 m^2$
B) $0.9 m^2$
C) $9 m^2$
D) $90 m^2$
E) $900 m^2$

END OF SECTION

Section 2

Question 23:
GLUT2 is an essential, ATP independent, mediator in the liver's uptake of plasma glucose. This is an example of:

A) Active transport
B) Diffusion
C) Exocytosis
D) Facilitated Diffusion
E) Osmosis

Question 24:
Which of the following cell types will have the greatest flux along endocytotic pathways?

A) Kidney cells
B) Liver cells
C) Nerve cells
D) Red blood cells
E) White blood cell

Question 25:
Compared to the Krebs cycle, the Calvin cycle demonstrates which of the following differences?

A) CO_2 as a substrate rather than a product
B) Photon dependent
C) Utilisation of different electron transporters
D) Net loss of ATP
E) All of the above

Question 26:
Pepsin and trypsin are both digestive enzymes. Pepsin acts in the stomach whereas trypsin is secreted by the pancreas. Which graph below (trypsin in black and pepsin in grey) would most accurately demonstrate their relative activity against pH?

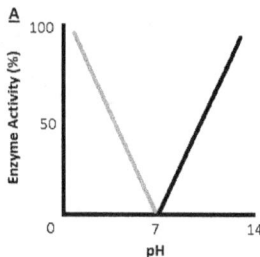
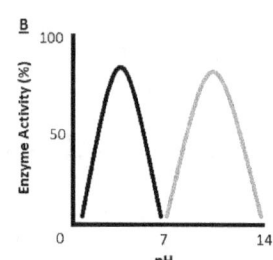
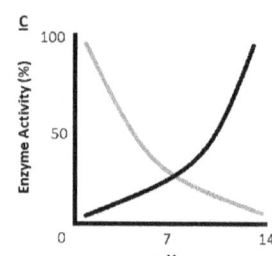
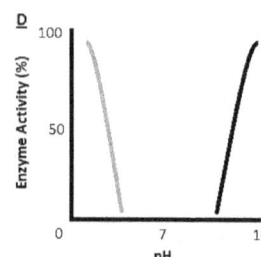
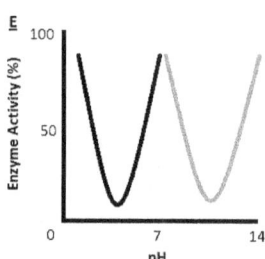

Question 27:
MRSA is an example of:

A) Natural selection
B) Genetic engineering
C) Sexual reproduction
D) Lamarckism
E) Co-dominance

Question 28:
Which of the following statements are correct regarding mitosis?

1. It is important in sexual reproduction.
2. A single round of mitosis results in the formation of 2 genetically distinct daughter cells.
3. Mitosis is vital for tissue growth, as it is the basis for cell multiplication.

A) Only 1
B) Only 2
C) Only 3
D) 1 and 2
E) 2 and 3
F) 1 and 3
G) 1, 2 and 3

Question 29:
Which of the following is the best definition of a mutation?

A) A mutation is a permanent change in DNA.
B) A mutation is a permanent change in DNA that is harmful to an organism.
C) A mutation is a permanent change in the structure of intra-cellular organelles caused by changes in DNA/RNA.
D) A mutation is a permanent change in chromosomal structure caused by DNA/RNA changes.

Question 30:
In relation to mutations, which of the following are correct?

1. Mutations always lead to discernible changes in the phenotype of an organism.
2. Mutations are central to natural processes such as evolution.
3. Mutations play a role in cancer.

A) Only 1
B) Only 2
C) Only 3
D) 1 and 2
E) 2 and 3
F) 1 and 3
G) 1, 2 and 3

Question 31:
Which of the following is the most accurate definition of an antibody?

A) An antibody is a molecule that protects red blood cells from changes in pH.
B) An antibody is a molecule produced only by humans and has a pivotal role in the immune system.
C) An antibody is a toxin produced by a pathogen to damage the host organism.
D) An antibody is a molecule that is used by the immune system to identify and neutralize foreign objects and molecules.
E) Antibodies are small proteins found in red blood cells that help increase oxygen carriage.

Question 32:
Which of the following statements about the kidney are correct?

1. The kidneys filter the blood and remove waste products from the body.
2. The kidneys are involved in the digestion of food.
3. In a healthy individual, the kidneys produce urine that contains high levels of glucose.

A) Only 1
B) Only 2
C) Only 3
D) 1 and 2
E) 2 and 3
F) 1 and 3
G) 1, 2 and 3

Question 33:
Which of the following statements are correct?

1. Hormones are slower acting than nerves.
2. Hormones act for a very short time.
3. Hormones act more generally than nerves.
4. Hormones are released when you get a scare.

A) 1 only
B) 1 and 3 only
C) 2 and 4 only
D) 1, 3 and 4 only
E) 1, 2, 3 and 4

Question 34:
Which statements about homeostasis are correct?

1. Homeostasis is about ensuring the inputs within your body exceed the outputs to maintain a constant internal environment.
2. Homeostasis is about ensuring the inputs within your body are less than the outputs to maintain a constant internal environment.
3. Homeostasis is about balancing the inputs within your body with the outputs to ensure your body fluctuates with the needs of the external environment.
4. Homeostasis is about balancing the inputs within your body with the outputs to maintain a constant internal environment.

A) 1 only   C) 3 only   E) 1 and 3 only   G) 2 and 3 only
B) 2 only   D) 4 only   F) 2 and 4 only

Question 35:

Which of the following statement is true?

A) There is more energy and biomass each time you move up a trophic level.
B) There is less energy and biomass each time you move up a trophic level.
C) There is more energy but less biomass each time you move up a trophic level.
D) There is less energy but more biomass each time you move up a trophic level.
E) There is no difference in the energy or biomass when you move up a trophic level.

Question 36:
Which of the following statements are true about asexual reproduction?

1. There is no fusion of gametes.
2. There are two parents.
3. There is no mixing of chromosomes.
4. There is genetic variation.

A) 1 and 3 only   C) 2 and 3 only   E) 2 and 4 only
B) 1 and 4 only   D) 3 and 4 only   F) 1, 2, 3 and 4

MOCK PAPER B — SECTION TWO

Question 37:
Put the following in the order which they occur when Jonas sees a bowl of chicken and moves towards it.

1. Retina
2. Motor neuron
3. Sensory neuron
4. Brain
5. Muscle

A) 1 - 3 - 4 - 5 - 2
B) 1 - 2 - 3 - 4 - 5
C) 5 - 1 - 3 - 2 - 4
D) 1 - 3 - 2 - 4 - 5
E) 1 - 3 - 4 - 2 - 5
F) 4 - 1 - 3 - 2 - 5

Question 38:
What path does blood take from the kidney to the liver?

1. Pulmonary artery
2. Inferior vena cava
3. Hepatic artery
4. Aorta
5. Pulmonary vein
6. Renal vein

A) 2 - 1 - 4 - 3 - 5 - 6
B) 1 - 2 - 3 - 4 - 5 - 6
C) 6 - 2 - 5 - 1 - 4 - 3
D) 6 - 2 - 1 - 5 - 4 - 3
E) 3 - 2 - 1 - 4 - 6 - 5
F) 3 - 6 - 2 - 4 - 1 - 5

Question 39:
Which of the following statements are true about animal cloning?

1. Animals cloned from embryo transplants are genetically identical.
2. The genetic material is removed from an unfertilised egg during adult cell cloning.
3. Cloning can cause a reduced gene pool.
4. Cloning is only possible with mammals.

A) 1 only
B) 2 only
C) 3 only
D) 4 only
E) 1 and 2 only
F) 1, 2 and 3 only
G) 1, 2, 3 and 4

Question 40:
Which of the following statements are true with regard to evolution?

1. Individuals within a species show variation because of differences in their genes.
2. Beneficial mutations will accumulate within a population.
3. Gene differences are caused by sexual reproduction and mutations.
4. Species with similar characteristics never have similar genes.

A) 1 only
B) 1 and 4 only
C) 2 and 3 only
D) 2 and 4 only
E) 3 and 4 only
F) 1, 2 and 3 only

END OF SECTION

Section 3

Question 41:
The molecular weight of glucose is 180 g/mol. 5.76Kg of glucose is split evenly between two cell cultures under anaerobic conditions. One cell culture is taken from human cardiac muscle, whilst the other is a yeast culture. What will be the difference (in moles) between the amount of CO_2 produced between the two cultures?

A) 0 mol   B) 4 mol   C) 8 mol   D) 12 mol   E) 16 mol

Question 42:
What is the electron configuration of magnesium in $MgCl_2$?

A) 2,8
B) 2,8,2
C) 2,8,4
D) 2,8,8
E) None of the above

Question 43:
A calcium sample is run in a mass spectrometer. It is later discovered that the sample was contaminated with the most abundant isotope of chromium. A section of the trace is shown below. What was the actual abundance of the most common calcium isotope?

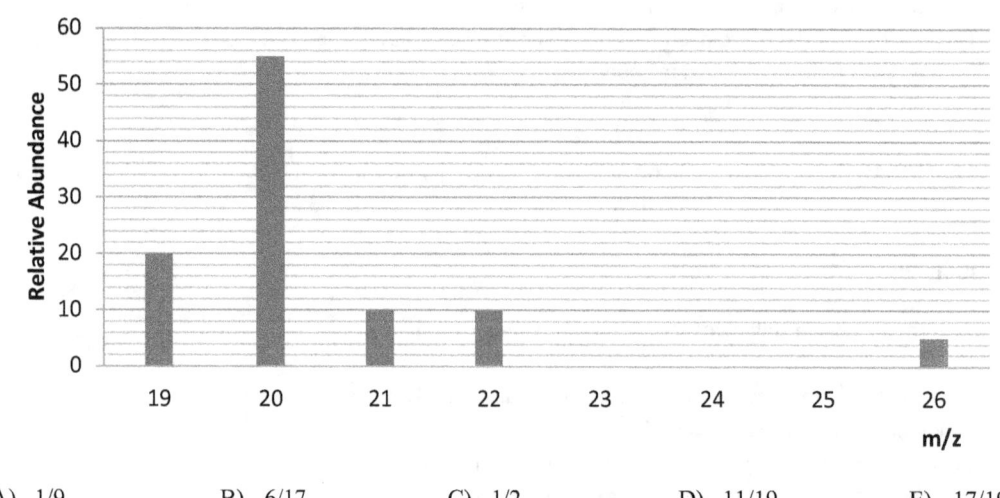

A) 1/9   B) 6/17   C) 1/2   D) 11/19   E) 17/19

Question 44:
A warehouse receives 15 tonnes of arsenic in bulk. Assuming that the sample is at least 80% pure, what is the minimum amount, in moles, of arsenic that they have obtained?

A) 1.6×10^5 B) 2×10^5 C) 1.6×10^6 D) 2×10^6 E) 1.6×10^7

Question 45:
A sample of silicon is run in a mass spectrometer. The resultant trace shows m/z peaks at 26 and 30 with relative abundance 60% and 30% respectively. What other isotope of silicon must have been in the sample to give an average atomic mass of 28?

A) 28   B) 30   C) 32   D) 34   E) 36

Question 46:
72.9g of pure magnesium ribbon is mixed in a reaction vessel with the equivalent of 54g of steam. The ensuing reaction produces 72dm³ of hydrogen. Which of the following statements is true?

A) This is a complete reaction
B) This is a partial reaction
C) There is an excess of steam
D) There is an excess of magnesium
E) Magnesium hydroxide is a product

Question 47:
Which species is the reducing agent in: $3Cu^{2+} + 3S^{2-} + 8H^+ + 8NO_3^- \rightarrow 3Cu^{2+} + 3SO_4^{2-} + 8NO + 4H_2O$

A) Cu^{2+} B) S^{2-} C) H^+ D) NO_3^- E) H_2O

Question 48:
Which of the following is not true of alkanes?

A) C_nH_{2n+2}
B) Saturated
C) Reactive
D) Produce only CO_2 and water when burnt in an excess of oxygen
E) None of the above

Question 49:
What values of **s, t** and **u** are needed to balance the equation below?
$sAgNO_3 + tK_3PO_4 \rightarrow 3Ag_3PO_4 + uKNO_3$

A) s = 9 t = 3 u = 9
B) s = 6 t = 3 u = 9
C) s = 9 t = 3 u = 6
D) s = 9 t = 6 u = 9
E) s = 3 t = 3 u = 9
F) s = 9 t = 3 u = 3

Question 50:
Which of the following statements are true with regard to displacement?

1. A less reactive halogen can displace a more reactive halogen.
2. Chlorine cannot displace bromine or iodine from an aqueous solution of its salts.
3. Bromine can displace iodine because of the trend of reactivity.
4. Fluorine can displace chlorine as it is higher up the group.
5. Lithium can displace francium as it is higher up the group.

A) 3 only
B) 5 only
C) 1 and 2 only
D) 3 and 4 only
E) 2, 3 and 5 only
F) 3, 4 and 5 only

Question 51:
What mass of magnesium oxide is produced when 75g of magnesium is burned in excess oxygen?
Relative Atomic Masses: Mg = 24, O = 16

A) 80g   B) 100g   C) 125g   D) 145g   E) 175g   F) 225g

Question 52:
Hydrogen can combine with hydroxide ions to produce water. Which process is involved in this?

A) Hydration
B) Oxidation
C) Reduction
D) Dehydration
E) Evaporation
F) Precipitation

END OF SECTION

Section 4

Question 53:
A rubber balloon is inflated and rubbed against a sample of animal fur for a period of 15 seconds. At the end of this process the balloon is carrying a charge of -5 coulombs. What magnitude of current must have been induced during the process of rubbing the balloon against the animal fur; and in which direction was it flowing?

A) 0.33A into the balloon
B) 0.33A into the fur
C) 0.33A in no net direction
D) 75A into the balloon
E) 75A into the fur

Question 54:
Which of the following is a unit equivalent to the Amp?

A) V.Ω B) (W.V)/s   C) C.Ω D) (J.s^{-1})/V   E) C.s

Question 55:
The output of a step-down transformer is measured at 24V and 10A. Given that the transformer is 80% efficient what must the initial power input have been?

A) 240W   B) 260W   C) 280W   D) 300W   E) 320W

Question 56:
An electric winch system hoists a mass of 20kg 30 metres into the air over a period of 20 seconds. What is the power output of the winch assuming the system is 100% efficient?

A) 100W   B) 200W   C) 300W   D) 400W   E) 500W

Question 57:
6 x 10^{10} atoms of a radioactive substance remain. The activity of the substance is quantified as 3.6 x 10^9. What is the decay constant of this material?

A) 0.00006   B) 0.0006   C) 0.006   D) 0.06   E) 0.6

Question 58:
An 80W filament bulb draws 0.5A of household electricity. What is the efficiency of the bulb?

A) 25%   B) 33%   C) 50%   D) 66%   E) 75%

Question 59:
An investment of £500 is made in a compound interest account. At the end of 3 years the balance reads £1687.50. What is the interest rate?

A) 20%   B) 35%   C) 50%   D) 65%   E) 80%

Question 60:

Rearrange the following equation in terms of t: $x = \frac{\sqrt{b^3 - 9st}}{13j} + \int_{-z}^{z} 9a - 7$

A) $t = \frac{(13jx - \int_{-z}^{z} 9a-7)^2 - b^3}{9s}$

B) $t = \frac{13jx^2}{b^3 - 9s} - \int_{-z}^{z} 9a - 7$

C) $t = x - \frac{\sqrt{b^3 - 9s}}{13j} - \int_{-z}^{z} 9a - 7$

D) $t = \frac{x^2}{\frac{b^3 - 9s}{13j} + \int_{-z}^{z} 9a - 7}$

E) $t = \frac{[13j(x - \int_{-z}^{z} 9a - 7)]^2 - b^3}{-9s}$

END OF PAPER

MOCK PAPER C

Section 1

Question 1:
Which US president was impeached in 1974?

A) Lyndon B Johnson
B) Richard Nixon
C) Gerald Ford
D) George Bush
E) Jimmy Carter

Question 2:
Which painter painted the Sistine chapel?

A) Leonardo Da Vinci
B) Michelangelo
C) Botticelli
D) Rembrandt
E) Gustav Klimt

Question 3:
The world's newest country succeeded in 2011, which is it?

A) South Sudan
B) Kosovo
C) Serbia
D) Norway
E) Fiji

Question 4:
Florence Nightingale first practiced nursing in which conflict?

A) WWI
B) WWII
C) The Crimea
D) The Napoleonic wars
E) The Boer War

Question 5:
Which of these writers was NOT a member of the Bloomsbury group?

A) Virginia Woolf
B) Lytton Strachey
C) E.M. Forster
D) John Maynard Keynes
E) Daniel Defoe

Question 6:
Which migratory bird has the largest known wingspan of up to 12 ft?

A) Flamingo
B) Canada Goose
C) Albatross
D) Great Blue Heron
E) American White Pelican

Question 7:

Which of these is not a real historical economic bubble?

A) The South Sea Bubble
B) The Tulip Bubble
C) The Housing Bubble
D) The Dot com Bubble
E) The Beer Bubble

Question 8:

Which piece of music was made to commemorate the Russian victory over Napoleon?

A) Holst's Jupiter
B) Tchaikovsky 1812 Overture
C) Stravinsky's Rites of Spring
D) Handel's Water music
E) Shostakovich' The Stalingrad symphony

Question 9:

In ancient Rome the so-called first triumvirate was made up of Julius Caesar, Crassus and who?

A) Marc Anthony
B) Cleopatra
C) Cicero
D) Pompey Magnus
E) Marcus Aurelius

Question 10:

Albert Einstein, Robert J. Oppenheimer and Ernest Lawrence were all scientist who worked on what together during WWII?

A) The Atomic bomb
B) Penicillin
C) The V-2 Bomb
D) Radar
E) The Helicopter

Question 11:

On 9/11 planes crashed into the World Trade Center in New York and what other building?

A) The Pentagon
B) The White house
C) The Empire State building
D) The Guggenheim
E) The Rockefeller Centre

Question 12:

Our Sun is what kind of star?

A) Red dwarf
B) White dwarf
C) Red giant
D) Blue giant
E) Yellow dwarf

Question 13:

Until the twentieth century, the whole purpose of art was to create beautiful, flawless works. Artists attained a level of skill and craft that took decades to perfect and could not be mirrored by those who had not taken great pains to master it. The serenity and beauty produced from movements such as impressionism has however culminated in repulsive and horrific displays of rotting carcasses designed to provoke an emotional response rather than admiration. These works cannot be described as beautiful by either the public or art critics. While these works may be engaging on an intellectual or academic level, they no longer constitute art.

Which of the following is an assumption of the above argument?

A) Beauty is a defining property of art.
B) All modern art is ugly.
C) Twenty first century artists do not study for decades.
D) The impressionist movement created beautiful works of art.
E) Some modern art provokes an emotional response.

Question 14:

The cost of sunglasses is reduced over the bank holiday weekend. On Saturday, the price of the sunglasses on Friday is reduced by 10%. On Sunday the price of the sunglasses on Saturday is reduced by 10%. On Monday, the price of the sunglasses on Sunday is reduced by a further 10%. What percentage of the price on Friday is the price of the sunglasses on Monday?

A) 55.12%   B) 59.10%   C) 63.80%   D) 70.34%   E) 72.9%

Question 15:
When folded, which box can be made from the net shown below?

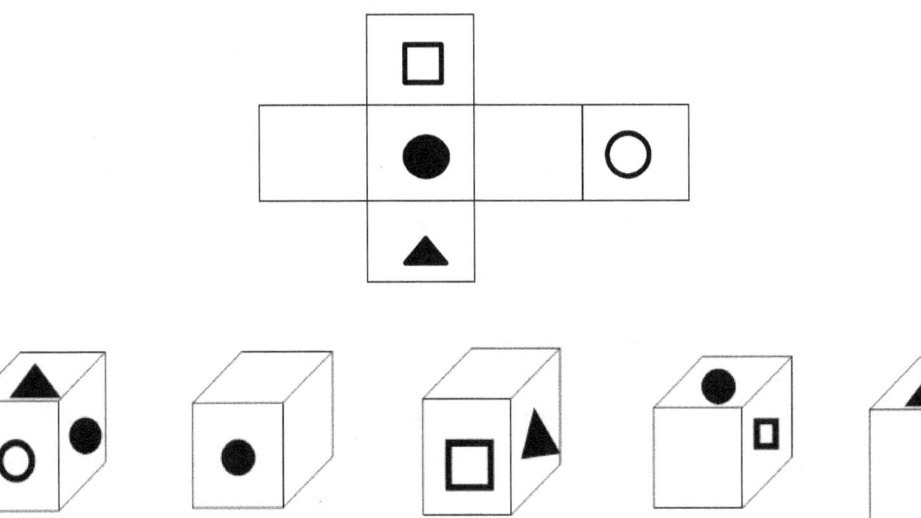

Questions 16-18 refer to the following information:

$$BMI = weight\ (kg) \div height^2\ (m^2)$$

Men	BMR= (10 x weight in kg) + (6.25 x height in cm) – (5 x age in years) + 5
Women	BMR= (10 x weight in kg) + (6.25 x height in cm) – (5 x age in years) -161

Recommended Intake:

Amount of Exercise	Daily Kilocalories required
Little to no exercise	BMR x 1.2
Light exercise 1-3 days per week	BMR x 1.375
Moderate exercise 3-5 days per week	BMR x 1.55
Heavy exercise 6-7 days per week	BMR x 1.725
Very heavy exercise twice per day	BMR x 1.9

Question 16:
A child weighs 35kg and is 120cm tall. What is the BMI of the child to the nearest two decimal places?

A) 0.0024   B) 24.28   C) 24.31   D) 42.01   E) 42.33

Question 17:
What is the BMR of a 32-year-old woman weighing 80kg and measuring 1.7m in height?

A) 643.7 kcal   B) 1537 kcal   C) 1541.5 kcal   D) 1707.5 kcal   E) 2707.5 kcal

Question 18:
What is the recommended intake of a 45-year-old man weighing 80kg and measuring 1.7m in height who does little to no exercise each week?

A) 1642.5 kcal   B) 1771.8 kcal   C) 1851 kcal   D) 1971 kcal   E) 2712.5 kcal

Question 19:
Putting the digit 7 on the right-hand side of a two-digit number causes the number to increase by 565. What is the value of the two-digit number?

A) 27 B) 52 C) 62 D) 66 E) 627

Question 20:
The grid is comprised of 49 squares. The shape's area is 588cm². What is its perimeter in cm?

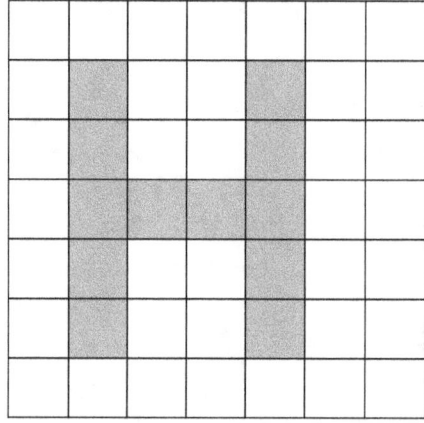

A) 26 B) 49 C) 84 D) 126 E) 182

Question 21:
Adam, Beth and Charlie are going on holiday together. A single room costs £60 per night, a double room costs £105 per night and a four-person room costs £215 per night. It is possible to opt out from the cleaning service and to pay £12 less each night per room.

What is the minimum amount the three friends could pay for their holiday for a three-night stay at the hotel?

A) £122 B) £144 C) £203 D) £423 E) £432

Question 22:
18 years ago, A was 25 years younger than B is now. In 21 years time, A will be 28 years older than B was 14 years ago. How old is A now if A is $\frac{5}{6}$B?

A) 27
B) 28
C) 35
D) 42
E) 46

END OF SECTION

Section 2

Question 23:
Which of the following statements regarding enzymes are correct?

1. Enzymes are denatured at high temperatures or extreme pH values.
2. Amylase is produced in the salivary glands only and converts starch to sugars.
3. Lipases catalyse the breakdown of oils and fats into glycerol and fatty acids. This takes place in the small intestine.
4. Bile is stored in the pancreas and travels down the bile duct to neutralise stomach acid.
5. Isomerase can be used to convert glucose into fructose for use in slimming products.

A) 1 and 3 only
B) 1, 3 and 4 only
C) 1, 3 and 5
D) 2 and 4 only
E) 3 and 5 only

Question 24:
Which of the following describes the role of the colon?

A) Food is combined with bile and digestive enzymes.
B) Storage of faeces.
C) Reabsorption of water.
D) Faeces leave the alimentary canal.
E) Any digested food is absorbed into the lymph and blood.

Question 25:
Which of the following are true?

1. A nerve impulse is transmitted along the nerve axon as an electrical impulse and across the synapse by diffusion of chemical neurotransmitters.
2. Drugs that block synaptic transmission can cause complete paralysis.
3. The fatty sheath around the axon slows the speed at which nerve impulses are transmitted.
4. The peripheral nervous system includes the brain and spinal cord.
5. A reflex arc bypasses the brain and enables a fast, autonomic response.

A) 1 and 2
B) 1, 2 and 3
C) 1, 2 and 5
D) 2, 4 and 5
E) 3, 4 and 5

Question 26:
Which of the following statements regarding the circulatory system are correct?

1. The pulmonary artery carries oxygenated blood from the right ventricle to the lungs.
2. The aorta has a high content of elastic tissue and carries oxygenated blood from the left ventricle around the body.
3. The mitral valve is between the pulmonary vein and the left atrium.
4. The vena cava carries deoxygenated blood from the body to the right atrium.

A) 1 and 3
B) 1 and 2
C) 2 only
D) 2 and 4
E) 3 only

MOCK PAPER C **SECTION TWO**

Question 27:
Tongue-rolling is controlled by the dominant allele T, while non-rolling is controlled by the recessive allele, t. Red-green colour blindness is controlled by a sex-linked gene on the X chromosome. Normal colour vision is controlled by dominant allele B, while red-green colour blindness is controlled by the recessive allele, b. The mother of a family is colour blind and heterozygous for tongue-rolling, while the father has normal colour vision and is a non-roller.

Which of the following statements are correct?

1. More males than females in a population are red-green colour blind.
2. 50% of children will be non-rollers.
3. All the male children will be colour-blind.

A) 1 and 2 only
B) 1, 2 and 3
C) 2 only
D) 2 and 3 only
E) 3 only

Question 28:
Which of the following are true?

1. Lightning, as well as nitrogen-fixing bacteria, converts nitrogen gas to nitrate compounds.
2. Decomposers return nitrogen to the soil as ammonia.
3. The shells of marine animals contain calcium carbonate, which is derived from dietary carbon.
4. Nitrogen is used to make the amino acids found in proteins.

A) 1 only
B) 1 and 2
C) 2 and 3
D) 2, 3 and 4
E) They are all true

Question 29:
Which of the following are correct regarding polymers?

1. Sucrose is formed by the condensation of hundreds of monosaccharides.
2. Lactose is found in milk and is formed by condensation of two glucose molecules.
3. Glucose has two isomers.
4. Glycogen, starch and cellulose are all polysaccharides formed by condensation of multiple glucose molecules.
5. People with lactose intolerance lack lactase and can experience diarrhoea after drinking milk.

A) 1 only
B) 1, 2 and 3
C) 1 and 3 only
D) 3, 4 and 5
E) 4 and 5 only

Question 30:
Which of the following genetic statements are correct?

1. Alleles are a similar version of different cells.
2. If you are homozygous for a trait, you have three alleles the same for that particular gene.
3. If you are heterozygous for a trait, you have two different alleles for that particular gene.
4. To show the characteristic that is caused by a recessive allele, both carried alleles for the gene have to be recessive.

A) 1 only
B) 2 only
C) 3 only
D) 4 only
E) 1 and 2 only
F) 3 and 4 only
G) 1, 2, and 3 only

Question 31:
Which of the following statements are correct about meiosis?

1. The DNA content of a gamete is half that of a human red blood cell.
2. Meiosis requires ATP.
3. Meiosis only takes place in reproductive tissue.
4. In meiosis, a diploid cell divides in such a way so as to produce two haploid cells.

A) 1 only
B) 3 only
C) 1 and 2 only
D) 2 and 3 only
E) 2 and 4 only
F) 1, 2, 3 and 4

Question 32:
Put the following statements in the correct order of events for when there is too little water in the blood.

1. Urine is more concentrated
2. Pituary gland releases ADH
3. Blood water level returns to normal
4. Hypothalamus detects too little water in blood
5. Kidney affects water level

A) 1 - 2 - 3 - 4 - 5
B) 5 - 4 - 3 - 2 - 1
C) 4 - 2 - 5 - 1 - 3
D) 3 - 2 - 4 - 1 - 5
E) 5 - 2 - 3 - 4 - 1
F) 4 - 2 – 1 - 5 - 3

Question 33:
The pH of venous blood is 7.35. Which of the following is the likely pH of arterial blood?

A) 4.4
B) 5.2
C) 6.5
D) 7.0
E) 7.4
F) 7.95

Question 34:
Which of the following are true of the cytoplasm?

1. The vast majority of the cytoplasm is made up of water.
2. All contents of animal cells are contained in the cytoplasm.
3. The cytoplasm contains electrolytes and proteins.

A) 1 only
B) 2 only
C) 3 only
D) 1 and 2 only
E) 1 and 3 only
F) 1, 2 and 3

Question 35:
ATP is produced in which of the following organelles?

1. The golgi apparatus
2. The rough endoplasmic reticulum
3. The mitochondria
4. The nucleus

A) 1 only
B) 2 only
C) 3 only
D) 4 only
E) 1 and 2
F) 2 and 3 only
G) 3 and 4 only
H) 1, 2, 3 and 4

Question 36:
The cell membrane:
A) Is made up of a phospholipid bilayer which only allows active transport across it.
B) Is not found in bacteria.
C) Is a semi-permeable barrier to ions and organic molecules.
D) Consists purely of enzymes.

Question 37:
Cells of the *Polyommatus atlantica* butterfly of the Lycaenidae family have 446 chromosomes. Which of the following statements about a *P. atlantica* butterfly are correct?

1. Mitosis will produce 2 daughter cells each with 223 pairs of chromosomes
2. Meiosis will produce 4 daughter cells each with 223 chromosomes
3. Mitosis will produce 4 daughter cells each with 446 chromosomes
4. Meiosis will produce 2 daughter cells each with 223 pairs of chromosomes

A) 1 and 2 only
B) 1 and 3 only
C) 2 and 3 only
D) 3 and 4 only
E) 1, 2 and 3 only
F) 1, 2, 3 and 4

Questions 38-40 are based on the following information:
Assume that hair colour is determined by a single allele. The R allele is dominant and results in black hair. The r allele is recessive for red hair. Mary (red hair) and Bob (black hair) are having a baby girl.

Question 38:
What is the probability that she will have red hair?

A) 0% only
B) 25% only
C) 50% only
D) 0% or 25%
E) 0% or 50%
F) 25% or 50%

Question 39:
Mary and Bob have a second child, Tim, who is born with red hair. What does this confirm about Bob?

A) Bob is heterozygous for the hair allele.
B) Bob is homozygous dominant for the hair allele.
C) Bob is homozygous recessive for the hair allele.
D) Bob does not have the hair allele.

Question 40:
Mary and Bob go on to have a third child. What are the chances that this child will be born homozygous for black hair?

A) 0%
B) 25%
C) 50%
D) 75%
E) 100%

END OF SECTION

Section 3

Question 41:
Which of the following statements are true regarding the transition elements?
1. Iron (II) compounds are light green.
2. Transition elements are neither malleable nor ductile.
3. Transition metal carbonates may undergo thermal decomposition.
4. Transition metal hydroxides are soluble in water.
5. When Cu^{2+} ions are mixed with sodium hydroxide solution, a blue precipitate is formed.

A) 1 and 2   B) 1 and 3   C) 1, 3 and 5   D) 3 and 5   E) 5 only

Question 42:
What is the value of C when the equation is balanced?

$\underline{5}$ PhCH$_3$ + $\underline{A}$ KMnO$_4$ + $\underline{9}$ H$_2$SO$_4$ = $\underline{5}$ PhCOOH + $\underline{B}$ K$_2$SO$_4$ + $\underline{C}$ MnSO$_4$ + $\underline{14}$ H$_2$O

A) 3   B) 4   C) 5   D) 7   E) 9

Question 43:
What is the mass in grams of calcium chloride, $CaCl_2$, in 25cm³ of a solution with a concentration of 0.1 mol.l⁻¹? (Ar of Ca is 40 and Ar of Cl is 35)

A) 0.28g   B) 0.46g   C) 0.48g   D) 0.72g   E) 1.28g

Question 44:
16.4g of nitrobenzene is produced from 13g of benzene in excess nitric acid: $C_6H_6 + HNO_3 \rightarrow C_6H_5NO_2 + H_2O$

What is the percentage yield of nitrobenzene ($C_6H_5NO_2$)?

A) 65%   B) 67%   C) 72%   D) 78%   E) 80%

Question 45:
Which of the following statements are false?
1. Simple molecules do not conduct electricity because there are no free electrons and there is no overall charge.
2. The carbon and silicon atoms in silica are arranged in a giant lattice structure and it has a very high melting point.
3. Ionic compounds do not conduct electricity when dissolved in water or when melted because the ions are too far apart.
4. Alloys are harder than pure metals.

A) 1 and 2   C) 1, 2, 3 and 4   E) 3 only

B) 1, 2 and 4   D) 2 and 4

Question 46:
A compound with a molar mass of 120 g.mol⁻¹ contains 12g of carbon, 2g of hydrogen and 16g oxygen. What is the molecular formula of the compound?

A) CH_2O B) $C_2H_4O_2$ C) C_4H_2O D) $C_4H_8O_4$ E) $C_8H_{16}O_8$

Question 47:
The following points refer to the halogens:

1. Iodine is a grey solid and can be used to sterilise wounds. It forms a purple vapour when warmed.
2. The melting and boiling points increase as you go up the group.
3. Fluorine is very dangerous and reacts instantly with iron wool, whereas iodine must be strongly heated as well as the iron wool for a reaction to occur and the reaction is slow.
4. When bromine is added to sodium chloride, the bromine displaces chlorine from sodium chloride.
5. The hydrogen atom and chlorine atom in hydrogen chloride are joined by a covalent bond.

Which of the above statements are false?

A) 1, 3 and 5
B) 1, 2 and 3
C) 2 and 4
D) 3 only
E) 3, 4 and 5

Question 48:
Which of the following statements about Ammonia are correct?

1. It has a formula of NH_3.
2. Nitrogen contributes 82% to its mass.
3. It can be broken down again into nitrogen and hydrogen.
4. It is covalently bonded.
5. It is used to make fertilisers.

A) 1 and 2 only
B) 1 and 4 only
C) 1, 2 and 3 only
D) 1, 2 and 5 only
E) 3, 4 and 5 only
F) 1, 2, 3, 4 and 5

Question 49:
What colour will a universal indicator change to in a solution of milk and lipase?

A) From green to orange.
B) From red to green.
C) From purple to green.
D) From purple to orange.
E) From yellow to purple.
F) From purple to red.

Question 50:
Vitamin C [$C_6H_8O_6$] can be artificially synthesised from glucose [$C_6H_{12}O_6$]. What type of reaction is this likely to be?

A) Dehydration
B) Hydration
C) Oxidation
D) Reduction
E) Displacement
F) Evaporation

Question 51:
Which of the following statements are true?

1. Cu^{64} will undergo oxidation faster than Cu^{65}.
2. Cu^{65} will undergo reduction faster than Cu^{64}.
3. Cu^{65} and Cu^{64} have the same number of electrons.

A) 1 only
B) 2 only
C) 3 only
D) 2 and 3 only
E) 1 and 3 only
F) 1, 2 and 3

Question 52:
6g of Mg^{24} is added to a solution containing 30g of dissolved sulphuric acid (H$_2$SO$_4$). Which of the following statements are true?
Relative Atomic Masses: S = 32, Mg = 24, O = 16, H = 1

1. In this reaction, the magnesium is the limiting reagent
2. In this reaction, sulphuric acid is the limiting reagent
3. The mass of salt produced equals the original mass of sulphuric acid

A) 1 only
B) 2 only
C) 3 only
D) 1 and 2 only
E) 1 and 3 only
F) 2 and 3 only

END OF SECTION

Section 4

Question 53:
Make y the subject of the formula: $\frac{y+x}{x} = \frac{x}{a} + \frac{a}{x}$

A) $y = \frac{x^2}{a} + a$

B) $y = \frac{x^2 + a^2 - ax}{a}$

C) $y = \frac{-ax}{x^2 + a^2}$

D) $y = \frac{x^2}{ax} + a - x$

E) $y = a^2 - ax$

Question 54:
Consider the equations: A: $y = 3x$ and B: $y = \frac{6}{x} - 7$. At what values of x do the two equations intersect?

A) x=2 and x=9
B) x=3 and x=6
C) x=6 and x=27
D) x=6
E) x=18

Question 55:
Rupert plays one game of tennis and one game of squash.
The probability that he will win the tennis game is $\frac{3}{4}$
The probability that he will win the squash game is $\frac{1}{3}$
What is the probability that he will win one game only?

A) $\frac{3}{12}$
B) $\frac{7}{12}$
C) $\frac{4}{5}$
D) $\frac{13}{12}$
E) $\frac{7}{6}$

Question 56:
What is the median of the following numbers: $\frac{7}{36}$; $0.\dot{3}$; $\frac{11}{18}$; 0.25; 0.75; $\frac{62}{72}$; $\frac{7}{7}$

A) $\frac{7}{36}$
B) $0.\dot{3}$
C) $\frac{11}{18}$
D) $\frac{62}{72}$
E) 0.75

Question 57:
Two carriages of a train collide and then start moving together in the same direction. Carriage 1 has mass 12,000 kg and moves at 5ms^{-1} before the collision. Carriage 2 has mass 8,000 kg and is stationary before the collision.
What is the velocity of the two carriages after the collision?

A) 2 ms^{-1}
B) 3 ms^{-1}
C) 4 ms^{-1}
D) 4.5 ms^{-1}
E) 5 ms^{-1}

MOCK PAPER C — SECTION FOUR

Question 58:
Which of the following points regarding electromagnetic waves are correct?

1. Radiowaves have the longest wavelength and the lowest frequency.
2. Infrared has a shorter wavelength than visible light and is used in optical fibre communication, and heater and night vision equipment.
3. All of the waves from gamma to radio waves travel at the speed of light (about 300,000,000 m/s).
4. Infrared radiation is used to sterilise food and to kill cancer cells.
5. Darker skins absorb more UV light, so less ultraviolet radiation reaches the deeper tissues.

A) 1 and 2
B) 1 and 3
C) 1, 3 and 5
D) 2 and 3
E) 2 and 4

Question 59:
Which of the following statements are true?

1. Control rods are used to absorb electrons in a nuclear reactor to control the chain reaction.
2. Nuclear fusion is commonly used as an energy source.
3. An alpha particle is comprised of two protons and two neutrons and is the same as a helium nucleus.
4. When $^{14}_{6}C$ undergoes beta decay, an electron and $^{14}_{7}N$ are produced.
5. Beta particles are less ionising than gamma rays and more ionising than alpha particles.

A) 1 and 2
B) 1 and 3
C) 3 and 4
D) 3, 4 and 5
E) None

Question 60:
Simplify fully: $\dfrac{(3x^{1/2})^3}{3x^2}$

A) $\dfrac{3x}{\sqrt{x}}$ B) $\dfrac{9}{x}$ C) $3x^{1/2}$ D) $3x\sqrt{x}$ E) $\dfrac{9}{\sqrt{x}}$

END OF PAPER

MOCK PAPER D

Section 1

Question 1:
The Mason and Dixon line, surveyed by Charles Mason and Jeremiah Dixon runs across which continent?

A) Asia
B) Africa
C) North America
D) South America
E) Europe

Question 2:
Franz Kafka lived in what central European Capital?

A) Berlin
B) Vienna
C) Budapest
D) Prague
E) Warsaw

Question 3:
Mansa Musa is sometimes considered to have been histories richest man, what empire did he rule?

A) Roman
B) Mongolian
C) Malian
D) Minoan
E) Japanese

Question 4:
Japan invaded what region of China during the early 20th century?
A) Tibet
B) Manchuria
C) Inner Mongolia
D) Guangxi
E) Xinjiang

Question 5:
In 1492 Isabella and Ferdinand united what country?
A) Portugal
B) Spain
C) Italy
D) Denmark
E) Norway

Question 6:
The what 'effect' is the change caused in a wavelength by the speed an observer is travelling?
A) Doppler effect
B) Mars effect
C) Hubble effect
D) Lambda effect
E) Euclid Effect

Question 7:
Which of these American cities was completely flooded during Hurricane Katrina?
A) New York
B) Chicago
C) San Francisco
D) New Orleans
E) Houston

Question 8:
In Law, to a commit a crime with Mens Rea means to commit a crime with what?
A) Intention
B) A weapon
C) Ignorance
D) Anger
E) Accomplices

Question 9:
The 2008 Olympic Games were held in what country?
A) Japan
B) USA
C) China
D) Italy
E) UK

Question 10:
In January 2018, scientists in China cloned the first what?
A) Pigs
B) Monkeys
C) Sheep
D) Dolphin
E) Cows

Question 11:
What American Author wrote the critically acclaimed novel *No Country for Old Men* in 2005?
A) Cormac McCarthy
B) Herman Melville
C) Toni Morrison
D) Thomas Pynchon
E) John Steinbeck

Question 12:
Newspeak is a word which comes from which book by George Orwell?
A) Nineteen Eighty Four
B) Down and Out in Paris and London
C) Homage to Catalonia
D) The Road to Wigan Pier
E) Animal Farm

Question 13:
"To make a cake you must prepare the ingredients and then bake it in the oven. You purchase the required ingredients from the shop, however your oven is broken. Therefore you cannot make a cake."

Which of the following arguments has the same structure?

A) To get a good job, you must have a strong CV then impress the recruiter at interview. Your CV was not as good as other applicants; therefore you didn't get the job.
B) To get to Paris, you must either fly or take the Eurostar. There are flight delays due to dense fog, therefore you must take the Eurostar.
C) To borrow a library book, you must go to the library and show your library card. At the library, you realise you have forgotten your library card. Therefore you cannot borrow a book.
D) To clean a bedroom window, you need a ladder and a hosepipe. Since you don't have the right equipment, you cannot clean the window.
E) Bears eat both fruit and fish. The river is frozen, so the bear cannot eat fish.

Question 14:
"Making model ships requires patience, skill and experience. Patience and skill without experience is common – but often such people give up prematurely, since skill without experience is insufficient to make model ships, and patience can quickly be exhausted."
Which of the following summarises the main argument?

A) Most people lack the skill needed to make model ships
B) Making model ships requires experience
C) The most important thing is to get experience
D) Most people make model ships for a short time but give up due to a lack of skill
E) Successful model ship makers need to have several positive traits

Question 15:
"Joseph has a bag of building blocks of various shapes and colours. Some of the cubic ones are black. Some of the black ones are pyramid shaped. All blue ones are cylindrical. There is a green one of each shape. There are some pink shapes."
Which of the following is definitely **NOT** true?

A) Joseph has pink cylindrical blocks
B) Joseph doesn't have pink cylindrical blocks
C) Joseph has blue cubic blocks
D) Joseph has a green pyramid
E) Joseph doesn't have a black sphere

Question 16:
A fair 6-faced die has 2 sides painted red. The die is rolled 3 times.
What is the probability that at least one red side has been rolled?

A) $8/27$ B) $19/27$ C) $21/27$ D) $24/27$ E) 1

Question 17:
"In a particular furniture warehouse, all chairs have four legs. No tables have five legs, nor do any have three. Beds have no less than four legs, but one bed has eight as they must have a multiple of four legs. Sofas have four or six legs. Wardrobes have an even number of legs, and sideboards have and odd number. No other furniture has legs. Brian picks a piece of furniture out, and it has six legs."

What can be deduced about this piece of furniture?
A) It is a table
B) It could be either a wardrobe or a sideboard
C) It must be either a table or a sofa
D) It must be either a table, a sofa or a wardrobe
E) It could be either a bed, a table or a sofa

Question 18:
Two friends live 42 miles away from each other. They walk at 3mph towards each other. One of them has a pet falcon which starts to fly at 18mph as soon as the friends set off. The falcon flies back and forth between the two friends until the friends meet. How many miles does the falcon travel in total?

A) 63   B) 84   C) 114   D) 126   E) 252

Question 19:
"Antibiotic resistance is on the increase. As a result, many antibiotics in our vast armoury are becoming ineffective against common infections. Probably the most significant contributor to this is the use of antibiotics in farming, as this exposes bacteria to antibiotics for no good reason, giving the opportunity for resistance to develop. If this worrying trend continues, we might, in 30 years time, be back in the Victorian situation, where people die from skin or chest infections we consider mild today."

Which of the following best represents the overall conclusion of the passage?

A) Antibiotic resistance is a serious issue
B) Antibiotics use in farming is essential
C) The use of antibiotics in farming could cause us serious harm
D) Victorians used to die from diseases we can treat today
E) Antibiotics can treat skin infections

Question 20:
A complete set of maths equipment includes a pen, a pencil, a geometry set and a pad of paper. Pens cost £1.50, pencils cost 50p, paper pads cost £1 and geometry sets cost £3. Sam, Dave and George each want complete sets, but Mr Browett persuades them to share some items. Sam and Dave agree to share a paper pad and a geometry set. George must have his own pen, but agrees that he and Sam can share a pencil.

What is the total amount spent?
A) £12.00
B) £13.50
C) £16.50
D) £17.50
E) £18.00

Question 21:
"Competitors need to be able to run 200 metres in under 25 seconds to qualify for a tournament. James, Steven and Joe are attempting to qualify. Steven and Joe run faster than James. James' best time over 200 metres is 26.2 seconds." Which response is definitely true?

A) Only Joe qualifies.
B) James does not qualify.
C) Joe and Steven both qualify.
D) Joe qualifies.
E) No one qualifies.

Question 22:
You spend £5.60 in total on a sandwich, a packet of crisps and a watermelon. The watermelon cost twice as much as the sandwich, and the sandwich cost twice the price of the crisps.
How much did the watermelon cost?

A) £1.20
B) £2.60
C) £2.80
D) £3.20
E) £3.60

END OF SECTION

Section 2

Question 23:
Which of the following is **NOT** present in the Bowman's capsule?

A) Urea
B) Glucose
C) Sodium
D) Water
E) Haemoglobin

Question 24:
The primary ions responsible for an action potential on a muscle cell membrane are Sodium and Potassium. Sodium concentration is higher than that of potassium outside the cell. Potassium concentration is higher than that of sodium inside the cell. Depolarisation occurs when the membrane potential increases (become more positive).

Which of the following **must** be true when a muscle cell membrane depolarises?

A) More potassium moves into the muscle cell than sodium.
B) More sodium moves into the muscle cell than potassium.
C) There is no net flow of sodium or potassium ions.
D) The membrane potential becomes more negative
E) None of the above

Question 25:
Which of the following in NOT a polymer?

A) Polythene
B) Glycogen
C) Collagen
D) Starch
E) DNA
F) Triglyceride

Question 26:
SIADH is a metabolic disorder caused by an excess of Anti-Diuretic Hormone (ADH) release by the posterior pituitary gland.

Which row best describes the urine produced by a patient with SIADH?

	Volume	Salt Concentration	Glucose
A)	High	Low	Low
B)	High	High	Low
C)	High	High	High
D)	Low	Low	Low
E)	Low	High	Low
F)	Low	High	High

Question 27:
The normal cardiac cycle has two phases, systole and diastole.

During diastole, which of the following is **FALSE**?
A) The aortic valve is closed
B) The ventricles are relaxing
C) There is blood in the ventricles
D) The pressure in the aorta increases
E) There is blood in the ventricles

Question 28:
Below is a graph showing the concentration of product over time as substrate concentration is increased. Some enzyme inhibitors are introduced.

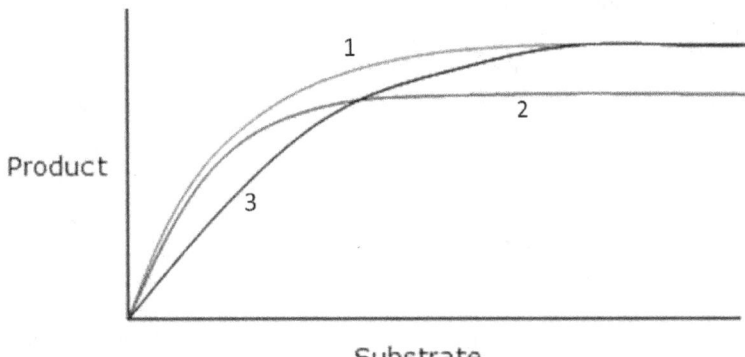

Which, if any, line represents the effect of competitive inhibition?

A) Line 1
B) Line 2
C) Line 3
D) None of these lines

Question 29:
Which of the following is **NOT** present in the plasma membrane?

A) Extrinsic proteins
B) Intrinsic proteins
C) Phospholipids
D) Glycoproteins
E) Nucleic Acids
F) They are all present

Question 30:
A pulmonary embolism occurs when a main artery supplying the lungs becomes blocked by a clot that has travelled from somewhere else in the body.

Which option best describes the path of a blood clot that originated in the leg and has caused a pulmonary embolism?

A. Inferior Vena cava
B. Superior Vena cava
C. Right atrium
D. Right ventricle
E. Left atrium
F. Left ventricle
G. Pulmonary artery
H. Pulmonary vein
I. Aorta
J. Coronary artery

A) C, D, H, G
B) B, C, D, H, G
C) I, E, F, G
D) A, C, D, G
E) A, C, D, J, G
F) A, C, D, J, E, F, G

Question 31:
The concentration of chloride in the blood is 100mM. The concentration of thyroxine is 1×10^{-10} kM. Calculate the ratio of thyroxine to chloride ions in the blood.

A) Chloride is 100,000,000 times more concentrated than thyroxine
B) Chloride is 1,000,000 times more concentrated than thyroxine
C) Chloride is 1000 times more concentrated than thyroxine
D) Concentrations of chloride and thyroxine are equal
E) Thyroxine is 1000 times more concentrated than chloride
F) Thyroxine is 1,000,000 times more concentrated than chloride

Question 32:
Which of the following is **NOT** a hormone?

A) Insulin
B) Glycogen
C) Noradrenaline
D) Cortisol
E) Thyroxine
F) Progesterone
G) None of the above

Question 33:
Which of the following statements regarding neural reflexes is **FALSE**?

A) Reflexes are usually faster than voluntary decisions
B) Reflex actions are faster than endocrine responses
C) The heat-withdrawal reflex is an example of a spinal reflex
D) Reflexes are completely unaffected by the brain
E) Reflexes are present in simple animals
F) Reflexes have both a sensory and motor component

Question 34:
The table below shows the results of a study investigating antibiotic resistance in staphylococcus populations.

Antibiotic	Number of Bacteria tested	Number of Resistant Bacteria
Benzyl-penicillin	10^{11}	98
Chloramphenicol	10^9	1200
Metronidazole	10^8	256
Erythtomycin	10^5	2

A single staphylococcus bacterium is chosen at random from a similar population. Resistance to any one antibiotic is independent of resistance to others.

Calculate the probability that the bacterium selected will be resistant to all four drugs.

A) 1 in 10^{12} B) 1 in 10^6 C) 1 in 10^{20} D) 1 in 10^{25} E) 1 in 10^{30} F) 1 in 10^{35}

Question 35:
Which of the following components of a food chain represent the largest biomass?

A) Producers
B) Decomposers
C) Primary consumers
D) Secondary consumers
E) Tertiary consumers

Question 36:
Why does air flow into the chest on inspiration?

1. Atmospheric pressure is smaller than intra-thoracic pressure during inspiration.
2. Atmospheric pressure is greater than intra-thoracic pressure during inspiration.
3. Anterior and lateral chest expansion decreases absolute intra-thoracic pressure.
4. Anterior and lateral chest expansion increases absolute intra-thoracic pressure.

A) 1 only
B) 2 only
C) 2 and 3
D) 1 and 4
E) 1 and 3
F) 2 and 4

Question 37:
Concerning the nitrogen cycle, which of the following are true?

1. The majority of the Earth's atmosphere is nitrogen.
2. Most of the nitrogen in the Earth's atmosphere is inert.
3. Bacteria are essential for nitrogen fixation.
4. Nitrogen fixation occurs during lightning strikes.

A) 1 and 2
B) 1 and 3
C) 2 and 3
D) 2 and 4
E) 3 and 4
F) 1, 2, 3 and 4

Question 38:
Which of the following statement are correct regarding mutations?

1. Mutations always cause proteins to lose their function.
2. Mutations always change the structure of the protein encoded by the affected gene.
3. Mutations always result in cancer.

A) Only 1
B) Only 2
C) Only 3
D) 1 and 2
E) 2 and 3
F) 1 and 3
G) 1, 2 and 3
H) None of the above

Question 39:
Which of the following is not a function of the central nervous system?

A) Coordination of movement
B) Decision making and executive functions
C) Control of heart rate
D) Cognition
E) Memory

Question 40:
Which of the following control mechanisms are involved in modulating cardiac output?

1. Voluntary control.
2. Sympathetic control to decrease heart rate.
3. Parasympathetic control to increase heart rate.

A) Only 1
B) Only 2
C) Only 3
D) 1 and 2
E) 2 and 3
F) 1 and 3
G) 1, 2 and 3
H) None of the above

END OF SECTION

Section 3

Question 41:
Place the following substances in order from most to least reactive:
1. Sodium
2. Potassium
3. Aluminium
4. Zinc
5. Copper
6. Magnesium

A) 1 » 2 » 6 » 3 » 4 » 5
B) 1 » 2 » 6 » 3 » 5 » 4
C) 2 » 1 » 6 » 3 » 4 » 5
D) 2 » 1 » 6 » 3 » 5 » 4
E) 2 » 6 » 1 » 3 » 4 » 5

Question 42:
A cup has 144ml of pure deionised water. How many electrons are in the cup due to the water? [Avogadro Constant = 6×10^{23}]

A) 8.64×10^{24}
B) 8.64×10^{25}
C) 1.2×10^{24}
D) 4.8×10^{24}
E) 4.8×10^{25}

Question 43:
Steve's sports car requires 2.28kg of octane to travel to Pete's house 10 miles away. Calculate the mass of CO_2 produced during the journey.

A) 0.88 kg
B) 1.66 kg
C) 2.64 kg
D) 3.52 kg
E) 5.28 kg
F) 7.04 kg

Question 44:
In which of the following mixtures will a displacement reaction occur?

1. $Cu + 2AgNO_3$
2. $Cu + Fe(NO_3)_2$
3. $Ca + 2H_2O$
4. $Fe + Ca(OH)_2$

A) 1 only
B) 2 only
C) 3 only
D) 4 only
E) 1 and 2 only
F) 1 and 3 only
G) 1, 2 and 3
H) 1, 2, 3 and 4

Question 45:
Which of the following statements is true about the following chain of metals?

$Na \rightarrow Ca \rightarrow Mg \rightarrow Al \rightarrow Zn$
Moving from left to right:

1. The reactivity of the metals increases.
2. The likelihood of corrosion of the metals increases.
3. More energy is required to separate these metals from their ores.
4. The metals lose electrons more readily to form positive ions.

A) 1 and 2 only
B) 1 and 3 only
C) 2 and 3 only
D) 1 and 4 only
E) 2, 3 and 4 only
F) 1, 2, 3 and 4
G) None of the above

Question 46:
In which of the following mixtures will a displacement reaction occur?

1. $I_2 + 2KBr$
2. $Cl_2 + 2NaBr$
3. $Br_2 + 2KI$

A) 1 only
B) 2 only
C) 3 only
D) 1 and 2 only
E) 1 and 3 only
F) 2 and 3 only
G) 1, 2 and 3

Question 47:
Which of the following statements about Al and Cu are true?

1. Al is used to build aircraft because it is lightweight and resists corrosion.
2. Cu is used to build electrical wires because it is a good insulator.
3. Both Al and Cu are good conductors of heat.
4. Al is commonly alloyed with other metals to make coins.
5. Al is resistant to corrosion because of a thin layer of aluminium hydroxide on its surface.

A) 1 and 3 only
B) 1 and 4 only
C) 1, 3 and 5 only
D) 1, 3, 4, 5 only
E) 2, 4 and 5 only
F) 2, 3, 4, 5 only

Question 48:
21g of Li^7 reacts completely with excess water. Given that the molar gas volume is 24 dm^3 under the conditions, what is the volume of hydrogen produced?

A) 12 dm^3
B) 24 dm^3
C) 36 dm^3
D) 48 dm^3
E) 72 dm^3
F) 120 dm^3

Question 49:
Which of the following statements regarding bonding are true?

1. NaCl has stronger ionic bonds than $MgCl_2$
2. Transition metals are able to lose varying numbers of electrons to form multiple stable positive ions.
3. All covalently bonded structures have lower melting points than ionically bonded compounds.
4. All covalently bonded structures do not conduct electricity.

A) 1 only
B) 2 only
C) 3 only
D) 4 only
E) 1 and 2 only
F) 2 and 3 only
G) 3 and 4 only
H) 1, 2 and 4 only

Question 50:
Which of the following pairs have the same electronic configuration?

1. Li^+ and Na^+
2. Mg^{2+} and Ne
3. Na^{2+} and Ne
4. O^{2-} and a Carbon atom

A) 1 only
B) 1 and 2 only
C) 1 and 3 only
D) 2 and 3 only
E) 2 and 4 only
F) 1, 2, 3 and 4

Question 51:
Consider the following two equations:

        A. $C + O_2 \rightarrow CO_2$ $\Delta H = -394$ kJ per mole

        B. $CaCO_3 \rightarrow CaO + CO_2$ $\Delta H = +178$ kJ per mole

Which of the following statements are true?

1. Reaction A is exothermic and Reaction B is endothermic
2. CO_2 has less energy than C and O_2.
3. CaO is more stable than $CaCO_3$.

A) 1 only   C) 3 only   E) 1 and 3   G) 1, 2 and 3
B) 2 only   D) 1 and 2   F) 2 and 3

Question 52:
Which of the following are true of regarding the oxides formed by Na, Mg and Al?

1. All of the metals and their solid oxides conduct electricity.
2. MgO has stronger bonds than Na_2O.
3. Metals are extracted from their molten ores by fractional distillation.

A) 1 only   C) 3 only   E) 2 and 3 only
B) 2 only   D) 1 and 2 only   F) 1, 2 and 3

END OF SECTION

Section 4

Question 53:
Calculate the radius of a sphere which has a surface area three times as great as its volume.

A) 0.5
B) 1
C) 1.5
D) 2
E) 2.5
F) More information is needed

Question 54:
A mechanical winch lifts up a bag of grain in a mill from the floor into a hopper.
Assuming that the machine is 100% efficient and lifts the bag vertically only, which of the following statements are **TRUE**?
1. This increases gravitational potential energy
2. The gravitational potential energy is independent of the mass of the grain
3. The work done is the difference between the gravitational potential energy at the hopper and when the grain is on the floor
4. The work done is the difference between the kinetic energy of the grain in the hopper and on the floor

A) 1 only
B) 1 and 3
C) 1 and 4
D) 1, 2 and 3
E) 1, 2 and 4
F) None of the above

Question 55:
A barometer records atmospheric pressure as 10^5 Pa. Recalling that the diameter of the Earth is 1.2 x 10^7 m, **estimate** the mass of the atmosphere. [Assume g = 10 ms^{-2}, the earth is spherical and that $\pi=3$]

A) 4.5 x 10^8 kg
B) 4.5 x 10^{10} kg
C) 4.5 x 10^{12} kg
D) 4.5 x 10^{13} kg
E) 4.5 x 10^{18} kg
F) More information is required

Question 56:
A 6kg missile is fired and decelerates at 6ms^{-2}.
What is the difference in resistive force compared to a 2kg missile fired and decelerating at 8ms^{-2}?

A) 8N
B) 12N
C) 16N
D) 20N
E) 24N

Question 57:
There are 1000 international airports in the world. If 4 flights take off every hour from each airport, estimate the annual number of commercial flights worldwide, to the nearest 1 million.

A) 20 million
B) 35 million
C) 37 million
D) 40 million
E) 42 million
F) 44 million

Question 58:
The figure below shows a schematic of a wiring system. All the bulbs have equal resistance. The power supply is 24V.

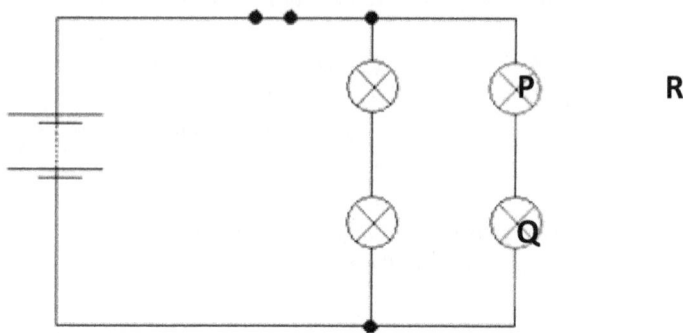

If headlight Q is replaced by a new one with twice the resistance, with the switch closed, which of these combinations of voltage drop across the four bulbs is possible?

	P	Q	R	S
A)	8V	16V	12V	12V
B)	8V	16V	16V	8V
C)	8V	16V	8V	16V
D)	12V	24V	24V	24V
E)	12V	12V	12V	12V
F)	16V	8V	12V	12V
G)	16V	8V	8V	16V
H)	24V	24V	24V	24V
I)	4V	8V	6V	6V
J)	8V	4V	6V	6V

Question 59:
Given:
F + G + H = 1
F + G − H = 2
F − G − H = 3

Calculate the value of FGH.

A) −2 B) −0.5 C) 0 D) 0.5 E) 2

Question 60:
Put the following types of electromagnetic waves in ascending order of wavelength:

	Shortest			Longest
A)	Visible Light	Ultraviolet	Infrared	X Ray
B)	Visible Light	Infrared	Ultraviolet	X Ray
C)	Infrared	Visible Light	Ultraviolet	X Ray
D)	Infrared	Visible Light	X Ray	Ultraviolet
E)	X Ray	Ultraviolet	Visible Light	Infrared
F)	X Ray	Ultraviolet	Infrared	Visible Light
G)	Ultraviolet	X Ray	Visible Light	Infrared

END OF PAPER

ANSWERS

ANSWER KEY

PAPER A

Section 1		Section 2		Section 3		Section 4	
1	A	23	A	41	E	53	B
2	B	24	E	42	D	54	D
3	A	25	D	43	B	55	B
4	B	26	B	44	E	56	C
5	E	27	D	45	D	57	A
6	C	28	D	46	C	58	C
7	C	29	A	47	B	59	B
8	B	30	F	48	A	60	C
9	E	31	F	49	E		
10	A	32	A	50	D		
11	A	33	C	51	E		
12	C	34	C	52	A		
13	E	35	D				
14	A	36	B				
15	D	37	A				
16	B	38	D				
17	C	39	D				
18	B	40	A				
19	D						
20	E						
21	C						
22	B						

PAPER B

Section 1		Section 2		Section 3		Section 4	
1	E	23	D	41	E	53	A
2	E	24	E	42	A	54	D
3	D	25	E	43	D	55	D
4	C	26	D	44	A	56	C
5	D	27	A	45	D	57	D
6	C	28	C	46	A	58	D
7	C	29	A	47	B	59	C
8	E	30	E	48	C	60	E
9	E	31	D	49	A		
10	E	32	A	50	D		
11	A	33	D	51	C		
12	C	34	D	52	B		
13	A	35	B				
14	D	36	A				
15	E	37	E				
16	B	38	D				
17	A	39	F				
18	B	40	F				
19	E						
20	E						
21	B						
22	A						

PAPER C

Section 1		Section 2		Section 3		Section 4	
1	B	23	C	41	C	53	B
2	B	24	C	42	E	54	C
3	A	25	C	43	A	55	B
4	C	26	D	44	E	56	C
5	E	27	B	45	E	57	B
6	C	28	E	46	D	58	C
7	E	29	D	47	C	59	C
8	B	30	F	48	F	60	E
9	D	31	D	49	A		
10	A	32	C	50	C		
11	A	33	E	51	C		
12	E	34	E	52	E		
13	A	35	C				
14	E	36	C				
15	E	37	A				
16	E	38	E				
17	C	39	A				
18	D	40	A				
19	C						
20	B						
21	D						
22	C						

PAPER D

Section 1		Section 2		Section 3		Section 4	
1	C	23	E	41	C	53	B
2	D	24	B	42	E	54	B
3	C	25	F	43	F	55	E
4	B	26	E	44	F	56	D
5	B	27	D	45	G	57	B
6	A	28	B	46	F	58	A
7	D	29	E	47	A	59	D
8	A	30	D	48	C	60	E
9	C	31	B	49	B		
10	B	32	B	50	D		
11	A	33	D	51	B		
12	A	34	D	52	E		
13	C	35	A				
14	E	36	C				
15	C	37	F				
16	B	38	H				
17	D	39	C				
18	D	40	H				
19	C						
20	B						
21	B						
22	A						

Mock Paper A Answers

Question 1: A
The Dolomite mountain range is located in South-Eastern Italy, part of the Southern Limestone Alps.

Question 2: B
The Marriage of Figaro is an Opera by Amadeus Mozart who lived in the 18th century. Of the other possible answers, only Beethoven was Mozart's contemporary. Chopin, Rimsky-Korsakov and Tchaikovsky are all 19th century composers.

Question 3: A
The Aztec Capital of Tenochtitlan, once the largest city on earth, was in what is now Mexico. The Mayans were also in Southern Mexico, and Central America. The Inca were based in Peru.

Question 4: B
Vermeer painted the girl with a Pearl Earring. Only Vermeer, Rembrandt and Van Gough were Dutch. Vermeer and Rembrandt were contemporaries during the Dutch Golden Age.

Question 5: E
This great speech is spoken by Marc Anthony at Caesar's funeral in Julius Caesar. The speech is meant to antagonise a crowd of onlookers against Caesar's murderers.

Question 6: C
Charlemagne united large parts of France, Germany and Northern Italy, and then had himself declared Emperor of the Romans by the pope, on Christmas day in 800 AD. Of the possible answers only Charles the Bald was also a Holy Roman Emperor.

Question 7: C
The Harlem Renaissance was an African-American artistic movement, Harlem is a borough of New York city.

Question 8: B
The Knights Hospitalier, also known as the Knights of St John, ruled Malta. Cyprus was briefly ruled by the Knights Templar, another chivalric order, whose job of protecting pilgrims had become defunct.

Question 9: E
Margaret Thatcher resigned in 1990, John Major was her successor.

Question 10: A
Io and Europa are two of Jupiter's many moons. They are, along with many of Jupiter's other moons, named after the deity's various lovers.

Question 11: A
FARC a Marxist movement formed during the cold war. The Shining Path are also a Marxists Latin American Group, based in Peru. ETA is a Basque separatist movement.

Question 12: C
The Metamorphoses was written by Ovid; Ovid, Virgil and Horace were all part of the Golden Age of Latin literature. Virgil was his contemporary and wrote the Aenied. Horace wrote various Odes and Satires. Dante was writing in Medieval Italy and Homer, if he really existed, was Greek.

Question 13: E
The question can be expressed as $(40 \times 30) - x(50 \times 30) = 200 = 1{,}200 - x1{,}500$. Therefore $x = 2/3$.

ANSWERS MOCK PAPER A

Question 14: A
As the largest digit on the number pad is 9, even if 9 was pressed for an infinitely long time the entered code would still average out at no larger than 9. Therefore, it would be impossible to achieve a reference number larger than 9. Indeed, this is an extremely insecure safe but not for the reason described in B (for if the same incorrect number was pressed indefinitely it would never average out as the correct one) but rather because the safe could in theory be opened with a single digit.

Question 15: D
A is incorrect as it ignores the section of the text that states the evolution of resistant strains is driven by the presence of antibiotics themselves. The text states that the rate of bacterial reproduction is a large contributing factor and therefore not wholly responsible – hence B is incorrect. Since this is just one example (and only the information in the text should be considered for these questions) for C to make such a general statement is complete unjustified.

Question 16: B
The fastest way to solve this question is to calculate the quantity of cheese per portion as 200/10 = 20. Which for 350 people would require 350 x 20 = 7000g or 7kg.

Question 17: C
Calculate the calorific content of 12 portions as 12 x 300 = 3,600kcal. As this represents 120%, evaluate what the initial amount would be as (3,600/120) x100 = 3,000kcal.

Question 18: B
Begin by calculating the initial weight of all the ingredients in the Bolognese sauce which comes to a total of 3.05kg. Therefore when cooking for 10 people 3.05 x 4 = 12.2kg of pasta should be used. Which in turn means for 30 people 3 x 12.2 = 36.6kg should be used.

Question 19: D
Calculate the new weight of ingredients in the Bolognese sauce excluding garlic and pancetta which produces a total of 2.8kg. Note that onions represent 0.3kg per 10 people and as such the ratio can be represented as 0.3/2.8 or alternatively dividing top and bottom by 0.3 → 1/9.3

Question 20: E
Begin with calculating total preparation time as 25 x 4 = 100 mins. The fact that Simon can only cook 8 portions at a time is somewhat a red herring as it doesn't impact the calculation. Total cooking time can be calculated as a further 25 x 8 = 200 mins. Producing a total time of 300mins or 5 hours.

Question 21: C
The simplest solution is to calculate the total area at the start as 20 x 20 = 400cm^2. Then recognise that with every fold the area will be reduced by half therefore the area will decrease as follows: 400, 200, 100, 50, 25, 12.5 – requiring a total of 5 folds.

Question 22: B
Off the 50% carrying the parasite 20% are symptomatic. Therefore 0.5 x 0.2 = 10% of the total population are infected and symptomatic. Of which 0.1 x 0.9 = 9% are male.

Question 23: A
An organ is defined as comprising multiple tissue types. As blood and skeletal muscle are themselves tissues they cannot be classified as organs.

ANSWERS MOCK PAPER A

Question 24: E
This question is best considered in terms of the aerobic respiration equation. With that in mind it becomes apparent that increased forward drive through the reaction will produce large amounts of water and CO_2 whilst demanding an increased supply of O_2. Further from this equation we realise that aerobic respiration produces large amounts of heat, and as such it is expected – in the interest of thermoregulation – that the body will both perspire and vasodilate in attempt to increase heat loss. Therefore, E is the correct answer.

Question 25: D
Recall that the nephron is the smallest functional unit of the kidney. The question therefore is asking you what is the smallest basic functional unit of striated muscle? To which the answer is the sarcomere. Note that a myofibril is a collection of many sarcomeres and is therefore not the correct answer.

Question 26: B
Insulin is a polypeptide hormone released by the pancreas in response to elevated plasma glucose levels. Therefore, it can be expected that plasma glucose concentration will be proportional to the concentration of insulin in the blood. Furthermore, recall that glucagon also released by the pancreas mobilises glucose stores. Therefore, the greatest concentration of plasma glucose would be expected at the time when glucagon is highest during a period of elevated insulin.

Question 27: D
Answers a and c are both nonsense and can be eliminated straight away. You will know from your study of the immune system that it is plasma B cells that produce antibodies and that plasma T cells do not exist. Also recall that an immune response can be mounted as quickly as within a fortnight which leaves the only correct answer d. The passage states that only once blood types are mixed is the immune response initiated, therefore answer d provides an explanation as to how this happens but also why the first-born child is unaffected.

Question 28: D
An organ consists of many cell types which once differentiated are committed to that single cell line. Therefore, a totipotent stem cell is required to produce the multiple cell types required. In order to ensure that the organ is an exact genetic match, stem cells from the individual in question must be used. Unless that individual is an embryo, adult stem cells must be used

Question 29: A
DNA consists of 4 bases: adenine, guanine, thymine and cysteine. The sugar backbone consists of deoxyribose, hence the name DNA. DNA is found in the cytoplasm of prokaryotes

Question 30: F
Mitochondria are responsible for energy production by ATP synthesis. Animal cells do not have a cell wall, only a cell membrane. The endoplasmic reticulum is important in protein synthesis, as this is where the proteins are assembled.

Question 31: F
If you aren't studying A-level biology, this question may stretch you. However, it is possible to reach an answer by process of elimination. Mitochondria are the 'powerhouse' of the cell in aerobic respiration, responsible for cell energy production rather than DNA replication or protein synthesis. As energy producers they are required in muscle cells in large numbers, and in sperm cells to drive the tail responsible for movement. They are enveloped by a double membrane, possibly because they started out as independent prokaryotes engulfed by eukaryotic cells.

Question 32: A
The majority of bacteria are commensals and don't lead to disease.

Question 33: C
Bacteria carry genetic information on plasmids and not in nuclei like animal cells. They don't need meiosis for replication, as they do not require gametes. Bacterial genomes consist of DNA, just like animal cells.

ANSWERS MOCK PAPER A

Question 34: C
Active transport requires a transport protein and ATP, as work is being done against an electrochemical gradient. Unlike diffusion, the relative concentrations of the materials being transported aren't important.

Question 35: D
Meiosis produces haploid gametes. This allows for fusion of 2 gametes to reach a full diploid set of chromosomes again in the zygote.

Question 36: B
Mendelian inheritance separates traits into dominant or recessive. It applies to all sexually reproducing organisms. Don't get confused by statement C – the offspring of 2 heterozygotes has a 25% chance of expressing a recessive trait, but it will be homozygous recessive.

Question 37: A
Hormones are released into the bloodstream and act on receptors in different organs in order to cause relatively slow changes to the body's physiology. Hormones frequently interact with the nervous system, e.g. Adrenaline and Insulin, however, they don't directly cause muscles to contract. Almost all hormones are synthesised.

Question 38 D
Neuronal signalling can happen via direct electrical stimulation of nerves or via chemical stimulation of synapses which produces a current that travels along the nerves. Electrical synapses are very rare in mammals, the majority of mammalian synapses are chemical.

Question 39: D
Remember that pH changes cause changes in electrical charge on proteins (= polypeptides) that could interfere with protein – protein interactions. Whilst the other statements are all correct to a certain extent, they are the downstream effects of what would happen if enzymes (which are also proteins) didn't work.

Question 40: A
The bacterial cell wall is made up of murein and protects the bacterium from the external environment, in particular from osmotic stresses, and is important in most bacteria.

Question 41: E
Recall that pH is a logarithmic scale of proton concentration and therefore will have the largest effect on hydrogen bonding.

Question 42: D
Isotopes of an element all contain the same number of protons but a different number of neutrons. As atomic number refers solely to the number of protons it will not change. However as mass number is the sum of atomic number and neutron number – it would be expected to change. If an isotope contains one extra proton, then assuming that the charge of that isotope is 0, then it must also contain one extra electron. Chemical properties are the same for all isotopes. Therefore, the correct answer is D.

Question 43: B
The transition metals are the most abundant catalysts – presumably due to their ability to achieve a variable number of stable states. Therefore, the correct answer is the d-block elements.

Question 44: E
Begin by writing down the balanced equation that describes the reaction of francium with water: $2Fr + 2H_2O \rightarrow 2FrOH + H_2$. Next calculate the moles of francium entering the reaction as $1338/223 = 6$. We therefore know from the stoichiometry of the equation that this reaction will produce 3 moles of hydrogen. Recall that 1 mole of gas at room temperature and pressure occupies $24dm^3$. Therefore, the hydrogen produced in this reaction will occupy $3 \times 24 = 72dm^3$.

ANSWERS **MOCK PAPER A**

Question 45: D
The simplest way to approach this type of question is to assume that there are 10 atoms within the compound. In this case that produces the following result: $C_3H_4F_2Cl$. Next look to see if any of the subscript numbers are divisible by a common factor. Also, if there are any decimals, multiply up by a common factor until only integers are present. In this case the correct answer is achieved straight away.

Question 46: C
This question requires you to have a correct answer from the previous question, although these questions are unfair in the fact that this current question cannot be answered without success in the first part – there are always one or two of these per paper. Simply calculate the Mr of your empirical formula: 113.5. And then divide 340.5 by this: 340.5/113.5 = 3. Therefore, multiply your empirical formula up by a factor of 3.

Question 47: B
The calculation in this question is simple: concentration = mass/volume, what this question is really testing is the manipulation of unorthodox units. Begin by noting the use of g/dL in the final answers and therefore begin by converting the quantities in the question into these units. 1.2×10^{10} kg = 1.2×10^{13} grams and with 10 decilitres in a litre, 4×10^{12} L = 4×10^{13} dL. $\frac{(1.2 \times 10^{13})}{(4 \times 10^{13})} = 3 \times 10^{-1}$ g/dL.

Question 48: A
A catalyst is not essential for the progression of a chemical reaction, it only acts to lower the activation energy and therefore increase the likelihood and rate of reaction.

Question 49: E
Cationic surfactants represent a class of molecule that demonstrates both hydrophilic and hydrophobic domains. This allows it to act as an emulsifying agent which is particularly useful in the disruption of grease or lipid deposits. Therefore, cationic surfactants have applications in all of the products listed.

Question 50: D
Different isotopes are differentiated by the number of neutrons in the core. This gives them different molecular weights and different chemical properties with regards to stability. The number of protons defines each element, and the number of electrons its charge.

Question 51: E
A displacement reaction occurs when a more reactive element displaces a less reactive element in its compound. All 4 reactions are examples of displacement reactions as a less reactive element is being replaced by a more reactive one.

Question 52: A
There needs to be 3Ca, 12H, 14O and 2P on each side. Only option A satisfies this.

Question 53: B
Let tail = T, body and legs = B and head = H.
As described in the question H = T + 0.5B and B = T + H. We have already been told that T = 30Kg.
Therefore, substitute the second equation into the first as H = 30 + 0.5(30 + H).
Re-arranging reveals that -0.5H = 45Kg and therefore the weight of the head is 90Kg, the body and legs 120Kg and as we were told the tail weighs 30Kg. Thus, giving a total weight of 240Kg

Question 54: D
Recall that kinetic energy can be calculated as $E = 0.5mv^2$. Therefore, if mass remains constant it is the v^2 term that must be reduced to a sixteenth. In other words, $v^2 = 1/16$ and therefore the correct velocity is $1/4x$.

Question 55: B
Recall that V = E/Q; therefore, when substituting SI units into these equation it is discovered that V = J/C = JC^{-1}.

Question 56: C
Recall that voltmeters are always connected in parallel – and so that they don't draw any current from the circuit have an infinite resistance. Ammeters on the other hand are connected in series and therefore must not perturb the flow of given, meaning they have zero resistance.

Question 57: A
Much of the information in this question is not needed and is simply put there to distract you. This question can be most quickly solved using the equation F=ma or force = mass x acceleration. As object A is the only things moving in this scenario it is the only source of energy to be considered. Its mass will be the same before and after the collision and so we need only calculate the magnitude of retardation. Given as $(15 - 3)/0.5 = 24 ms^{-2}$. Therefore, when plugging into the first equation we realise that F = 12 x 24 = 288N of force dissipated. Alternatively, this question could be solved by calculating the rate of change of momentum.

Question 58: C
Note the atomic masses and numbers in the equation. Whilst the atomic mass has remained constant the atomic number has increased by one and hence the element has changed. The only explanation for this is that a neutron has turned into a proton (and an electron which is represented by x). Therefore, the correct answer is C – beta radioactive decay.

Question 59: B
Begin by calculating the velocity of the wave as speed = wavelength x frequency = 3 x 20 = 60km/s. Which in a time period of one hour (3600s) would equate to a total distance of 60 x 3600 = 216,000km.

Question 60: C
The numerator of the fraction consists of 3 distinct terms or 3 distinct dimensions. As all other functions within the equation are constants one would consider this the volume of a complex 3D shape.

END OF PAPER

Mock Paper B Answers

Question 1: E
Juno went into orbit around Jupiter. Juno was Jupiter's wife in Roman mythology.

Question 2: E
The Volta river, not to be confused with the Volga, runs through West Africa. The Danube runs through Central and Eastern Europe. The Elbe runs through Germany and Czech Republic. The Seine runs through France and the Rhine through Switzerland and Germany.

Question 3: D
The American declaration of Independence was signed in 1776. 1789 was the date of the French revolution; many French people were inspired by their American counterparts' break for freedom.

Question 4: C
Nelson Mandela was released from prison in 1990.

Question 5: D
Sometimes known as the Kyoto agreement, or Kyoto Protocol, signed in 1997 and implemented in 2005.

Question 6: C
Marie and her husband studied the effects of radiation, with disastrous personal consequences. She discovered both Radium and Polonium and won the Nobel prize twice for her work.

Question 7: C
Voltaire, who was widely known in Europe at the time for saying things that got him into trouble.

Question 8: E
Hungary was never part of Yugoslavia, many of its members were previously part of the Austro-Hungarian Empire.

Question 9: E
Clarissa was written by Samuel Richardson, not Jane Austen.

Question 10: E
Bastille day is the 14th of July, not long after American Independence Day, which is on July 4th.

Question 11: A
'Hell is other people' comes from Jean-Paul Sartres' play, No Exit, in which the characters' hell is to be trapped in a waiting room together for eternity. Of the other possible answers, only Albert Camus was a French existentialist writer, and he was by all accounts, less misanthropic.

Question 12: C
Siddhartha was the Buddha's original name as a prince living in Northern India before giving it all up to sit under the Bodhi tree.

Question 13: A
Begin by converting all the quantities into terms of items as that is the terminology used on the graph axis. Therefore 12 rugby balls = 6 items and 120 tennis balls = 24 items. Reading from the graph reveals their respective prices as £9 and £5. Therefore, the total cost of products in the order is (6 x 9) + (24 x 5) = 174. Since this is significantly more than £100 the delivery charge is waived.

ANSWERS MOCK PAPER B

Question 14: D
Calculate the cost of 10 of everything as (2 x 5) x (10 x 7) x (5 x 9) = £125. Recall that delivery charge is waived at £100 and this therefore a trick question and no delivery charge is applied anyway.

Question 15: E
Tennis balls are sold in the largest pack and so they must be considered. Begin by dividing 1000/5 using the value from the first column = 200. As this is above the range 0 -99 look up the item value in the 100 -499 range where a £1 discount is applied per item. Therefore, in actually fact 1000/4 = 250 items can be purchased which equates to a total of 250 x 5 = 1250 balls.

Question 16: B
Recognise that 120% profit is equivalent to 220% of the original price. In which case the initial purchase price = (1,320/220) x 100 = £600.

Question 17: A
Note that here the question uses the term item and therefore simply read the costs directly off the graph giving a total order cost of (2 x 2000) + (4 x 2000) + (6 x 2000) = 24,000. Recall though that he only pays tax on the amount over £12,000 which in this case is £12,000. Therefore, he pays 12,000/4 = £3,000 tax.

Question 18: B
Lucy must live between Vicky and Shannon. Lucy is Vicky's neighbour, so Shannon cannot have a red door. Vicky lives next to someone with a red door, so Lucy must have the red door. This leaves Shannon with the blue door and Lucy with the white. The green door is across the road and so does not belong to any of them.

Question 19: E
First calculate an average complete one-way journey time as 40 + 5 + 5 = 50 minutes. Deducting his breaks, he works a total of 7 hours 20 or 440 minutes. Since the first train is already loaded his first run will only take 45 minutes leaving 395 minutes to complete his working day. 395/50 = 7 remainder 45. Note that 45 minutes is not enough to fully unload the train, but it is enough to load the train and drive the distance. Therefore, the driver will complete a total of 9 journeys equalling a distance of 198 miles.

Question 20: E
A is not actually a valid assumption as we do not know what proposal conservationists might be bringing to the local councils, they have only expressed their concern. They may well be bringing a proposal to ask for funding to rehome all the species in the affected environment. B is essential to the final paragraph whilst C must be assumed otherwise the councils would not be presenting these proposals at all.

Question 21: B
Let my current age = m and my brother's current age = g. The first section of this question can therefore be expressed as $m + 4 = 1/3(g + 1)$ whereas the second half can be represented as $2(m + 20) = g + 20$. Therefore, this problem can be solved as simultaneous equations. Rearranged the second equation reads $m = 1/2g - 10$; when substituted into the first equation we form $1/2g – 10 + 4 = 1/3(g + 1)$. Expand and simplify to $1/2g – 6 = 1/3g + 1/3$ → $1/6g = 6\frac{1}{3}$ which therefore means my brother's current age = $6\frac{1}{3} / (1/6) = 114/3 = 38$. Which means that my current age = $1/2(38) – 10 = 9$.

Question 22: A
This question can be solved quickly if you first realise that there is no need to calculate both volumes and subtract the larger from the smaller, instead only convert the television dimensions into metres and then calculate 60% of that.

ANSWERS MOCK PAPER B

Question 23: D
As the question states that GLUT2 is ATP independent then answer A) active transport is instantly incorrect as it is ATP dependent. Osmosis is applicable only to water molecules and is therefore incorrect. Exocytosis refers to the movement of molecules out of a cell and is therefore incorrect. Simple diffusion is incorrect as the question states that GLUT2 is essential for the process. This leaves the correct answer of facilitated diffusion.

Question 24: E
Firstly, recall that endocytosis is a process of molecular transport into cells that result in vesicular formation. This question requires you to realise the special case of this which is phagocytosis – conducted by white blood cells in the ingestion of pathogens.

Question 25: E
All of the above statements are true of the Calvin cycle with regards to the Krebs cycle. As the main driver of photosynthesis, we know that the Calvin cycle requires both CO_2 and light in order to conduct ATP dependent reactions. As opposed to the Krebs cycle in man however, the Calvin cycle adopts the use of NADPH as the intermediate in electron transport.

Question 26: D
Option D is one of only 2 graphs that demonstrate a quadratic relationship with the peak enzyme activity correctly placed – pepsin from the stomach close to pH 1, and trypsin secreted by the pancreas and therefore alkaline around pH 13. The curves traced in option c however are far too broad over the pH range to represent enzyme activity. As the pH scale is logarithmic, even a change of 1 or 0.5 can be devastating to enzyme activity.

Question 27: A
This question was taken directly from the IMAT syllabus where many examples are listed for different principles. Reading the IMAT syllabus and highlighting these is a very good idea as well as learning the definitions listed.

Question 28: C
Sexual reproduction relies on formation of gametes during **meiosis**. Mitosis doesn't produce genetically distinct cells. Mitosis is, however, the basis for tissue growth.

Question 29: A
A mutation is a permanent change in the nucleotide sequence of DNA. Whilst mutations may lead to changes in organelles and chromosomes, or even be harmful, they are strictly defined as permanent changes to the DNA or RNA sequence.

Question 30: E
Mutations are fairly common, but in the vast majority of cases do not have any impact on phenotype due to the redundancy of the genome. Sometimes they can confer selective advantages and allow organisms to survive better (i.e. evolve by natural selection), or they can lead to cancers as cells start dividing uncontrollably.

Question 31: D
Antibodies represent a pivotal molecule of the immune system. They provide very pointed and selective targeting of pathogens and toxins without causing damage to the body's own cells.

Question 32: A
Kidneys are not involved in digestion, but do filter the blood of waste products. Glucose is found in high concentrations in the urine of diabetics, who cannot absorb it without working insulin.

Question 33: D
Hormones are slower acting than nerves and act for a longer time. Hormones also act in a more general way. Adrenaline is also a hormone released into the body causing the fight-or-flight response. Although it is quick acting, it still lasts for a longer time than a nervous response, as you can still feel its effects for a time after the response, e.g. shaking hands.

ANSWERS MOCK PAPER B

Question 34: D
Homeostasis is about minimising changes to the internal environment by modulating both input and output.

Question 35: B
There is less energy and biomass each time you move up a trophic level. Only 10% of consumed energy is transferred to the next trophic level, so only one tenth of the previous biomass can be sustained in the next trophic level up.

Question 36: A
In asexual reproduction, there is no fusion of gametes as the single parent cell divides. There is therefore no mixing of chromosomes and, as a result, no genetic variation.

Question 37: E
The image is first formed on the retina which conveys it to the brain via a sensory nerve. The brain then sends an impulse to the muscle via a motor neuron.

Question 38: D
Blood from the kidney returns to the heart via the renal (kidney-related) vein, which drains into the inferior vena cava. The blood then passes through the pulmonary vasculature (veins carry blood to the heart, arteries away from the heart) before going into the aorta and eventually the hepatic (liver-related) artery.

Question 39: F
Clones are genetically identical by definition, and a large number of them could conceivably reduce the gene pool of a population. In adult cell cloning, the genetic material of an egg is replaced with the genetic material of an adult cell. Cloning is possible for all DNA based life forms, including plants and other types of animals.

Question 40: F
Gene varieties cause intraspecies variation, e.g. different eye colours. If mutations confer a selective advantage, those individuals with the mutation will survive to reproduce and grow in numbers. Genetic variation is caused by mixing of parent genomes and mutations. Species with similar characteristics often do have similar genes.

Question 41: E
In order to answer this question you must recall that anaerobic respiration in humans produces only lactate and energy, whilst in yeast the anaerobic respiratory process yields a molecule of ethanol and CO_2 per glucose molecule. Therefore, there will be 0 mol of CO_2 produced in the human cell culture and you need only work out the moles of CO_2 produced by the yeast cell culture to calculate the difference. There is a total of $5.76/0.18 = 32$ mol of glucose, of which half is supplied to the yeast cell culture. With a stoichiometric ratio of 1:1 in the anaerobic respiration equation a total of 16 mol of CO_2 will be produced.

Question 42: A
Initially the electron configuration of Mg is 2,8,2. In binding to two chlorine atoms it is effectively ionised to Mg^{2+} and it loses two electrons to leave a complete outer shell and thus the correct answer is 2,8.

Question 43: D
The first thing to note in this trace is that the m/z axis has been cut short. From looking up the mass of calcium in the periodic table one would expect to see the x axis centred around 40. However here the trace is only displaying those isotopes with valence 2 ($z = 2$) hence the values are half the size. Therefore (from the periodic table) when dividing the most abundant isotope of chromium by two, $52/2 = 26$, we confirm that the outlier bar on the right is indeed the contaminant. Therefore, to calculate the actual abundance of Mr 40 calcium ignore the chromium like so: $55/95 = 11/19$.

Question 44: A
Begin by converting the total weight of arsenic into grams like so $15 \times 10^6 = 1.5 \times 10^7$. Then divide by the Mr of arsenic which is 75 (2sf) giving 2×10^5. Don't forget that the sample is at worst 80% pure. Therefore, there will be a minimum of $(2 \times 10^5) \times 0.8 = 1.4 \times 10^5$ moles of pure arsenic.

Question 45: D
Recall that average atomic mass is calculated as the sum of (isotope mass x relative abundance). Therefore 28 = (26 x 0.6) + (30 x 0.3) + 0.1x. Rearranging this equation reveals that 0.1x = 3.4 and that the mystery isotope therefore has an atomic mass of 34.

Question 46: A
First recall that when a group 2 metal is reacted with steam a metal oxide is formed and therefore the following chemical equation can be drawn: $Mg + H_2O_{(g)}$ → $MgO + H_2$. Note the stoichiometric ratio which is simply 1. Next calculate that there is 72/24 = 3 mol of hydrogen produced. Therefore, assuming that there is 3 mol of all other reactants and the reaction is complete one would expect 3 x 24.3 = 72.9g of magnesium and 3 x 18 = 54g of steam. This is indeed the case and therefore the reaction is complete.

Question 47: B
The reducing agent is the species which is itself reduced in this instance from looking at the oxidation states we can see that that species is S^{2-}. As after the reaction has taken place it has an oxidation state of +6 which would require a loss of negative charge i.e. electrons.

Question 48: C
The highly stable bonds between carbon atoms, and between carbon and hydrogen atoms renders alkanes relatively unreactive. This is important to note as it highlights the major difference between alkanes and alkenes.

Question 49: A
To balance the equation there needs to be 9Ag, 9N, 9O_3, 9K, 3P on each side. Only option A satisfies this.

Question 50: D
A more reactive halogen can displace a less reactive halogen. Thus, chlorine can displace bromine and iodine from an aqueous solution of its salts, and fluorine can replace chlorine. The trend is the opposite for alkali metals, where reactivity increases down the group as electrons are further from the core and easier to lose.

Question 51: C
$2Mg + O_2 = 2MgO$; so, 2 x 24 = 48 and 2 x (24 + 16) = 80; so, 48 g of magnesium produces 80g of magnesium oxide; so 1g of magnesium produces 1g x 80g/48g = 1.666g oxide; so 75g x 1.666 = 125g

Question 52: B
$H_2 + 2OH^-$ → $2H_2O + e^-$. Thus, the hydrogen loses electrons i.e. is oxidised.

Question 53: A
Recall that current = charge/time. The question provides both charge and time in the correct units and so the calculation is relatively simple with no unit conversions required. Therefore current = 5/15 = 1/3 = 0.33A. As the question states that the balloon has a negative charge it has therefore gained electrons. Given that a current is defined as a net movement of electrons, in this situation the current must be flowing into the balloon.

Question 54: D
Given that Power = IV it can be deduced that I = P/V. Recall that power given in Watts is a measure of the energy transferred per second and therefore has the alternative units Js^{-1}. When substituting these units into the power equation re-arranged for Amps it is revealed that I = (Js^{-1})/V = A.

Question 55: D
For a transformer that is 100% efficient power in must equal power out, recalling that P=IV. Therefore, the transformer has a power output of 24 x 10 = 240W which is 80% of the initial input. As such the initial power input was (240/80) x 100 = 300W.

Question 56: C
Begin by calculating the energy required to hoist the mass, this is calculated using the potential energy equation: mgh. Energy = mass x g x height = 20 x 10 x 30 = 6000N. The power output of the motor is calculated as the joules dissipated per second = 6000/20 = 300W

Question 57: D
In order to solve this problem recall that activity = decay constant x number of remaining atoms. Therefore, the decay constant can be calculated simply as 0.36/6 = 0.06.

Question 58: D
Recall that household electricity is available in the UK at 240V. Begin by calculating the wattage that the bulb is receiving as 0.5 x 240 = 120W. Given that the energy rating of the bulb is 80W, we can assume that this bulb is only 80/120 = 66% efficient.

Question 59: C
The formula for calculating compound interest can be given as investment x (interest rate^{years}) or in short hand for this situation: $1687.5 = 500x^3$. Therefore, in order to calculate the interest rate the above formula must be rearranged to $\sqrt[3]{1687.5/500} = 1.5$ revealing an interest rate of 50%.

Question 60: E
Begin by subtracting the integral from both sides producing $x - \int_{-z}^{z} 9a - 7 = \frac{\sqrt{b^3 - 9st}}{13j}$. Next multiply both sides by 13j and square, rendering $[13j(x - \int_{-z}^{z} 9a - 7)]^2 = b^3 - 9st$. Finally subtract b^3 from both sides and divide by -9s leaving the correct answer: $\frac{[13j(x - \int_{-z}^{z} 9a - 7)]^2 - b^3}{-9s} = t$.

END OF PAPER

Mock Paper C Answers

Question 1: B
Richard Nixon was impeached for spying on his political opponents, and unusually, getting caught.

Question 2: B
Bits of the Sistine Chapel were painted by multiple painters including Botticelli, Perugino and Ghirlandaio. The ceiling itself though, and the Creation of Adam, was painted by Michelangelo.

Question 3: A
Kosovo is the second youngest and was given independence from Serbia in 2008.

Question 4: C
Florence Nightingale volunteered to work during the Crimean war, where her practice came to be greatly admired.

Question 5: E
The Bloomsbury Group writers were all living in London in the Edwardian period and experimenting with new ideas. Daniel Defoe lived much earlier and was most famous for writing Robinson Crusoe.

Question 6: C

Although all large birds, the Albatross is the largest.

Question 7: E
The beer bubble is not a real bubble, although the craft beer market is rumoured to be oversaturated.

Question 8: B
The 1812 overture was written to celebrate the defeat of Napoleon in that year. The Stalingrad Symphony was given that title by the USSR, and declared a celebration of the troops who fought there in WWII.

Question 9: D
The first triumvirate was an alliance between Julius Caesar, Crassus and Pompey Magnus. Marc Anthony and Marcus Lepidus were members of the second Triumvirate, which formed after Julius Caesar's death.

Question 10: A
All these things were invented during WWII, but those scientists all worked on the Manhattan project specifically, to build the atomic bomb.

Question 11: A
A third plane crashed into the pentagon at the same time.

Question 12: E
Our sun is a yellow dwarf.

Question 13: A
The main conclusion is option A that some works of modern art no longer constitute art. B is not an assumption made by the author as the main conclusion does not rely on *all* modern art being ugly to be valid. C is not an assumption because the argument does not rely on artists studying for decades to produce pieces of work that constitute art. This point is simply used to support the main argument. Options D and E are stated in the argument so are not assumptions. A is an assumption because it is required to be true to support the main conclusion but is not explicitly stated in the argument.

ANSWERS MOCK PAPER C

Question 14: E
Reducing the price of the sunglasses by 10% is equivalent to multiplying the price by 0.9. the price of the sunglasses is successively reduced by 10% three times and so the price on Monday is 0.9^3 the price of the sunglasses on Friday. 0.9^3 is equal to 0.729 and so the price of the sunglasses on Monday is 72.9% of the price of the sunglasses on Friday.

Question 15: E
Look at the flat cube net and note the shapes that are adjacent to each other. Sides that are joining on the net will be beside each other on the formed cube. Work through to deduce option E can be formed from the cube net shown.

Question 16: E
The information provided about the child needs to be inserted into the BMI formula: BMI=$35 \div 1.2^2$
1.2 squared is equal to 1.44 and it may be easier to work out 3500 divided by 144. The answer needs to be worked out to 3 decimal places for an answer required to 2 decimal places. The answer to 3 decimal places is 24.305 and so the BMI to 2 decimal places is 24.31.

Question 17: C
It is important that the information is inserted into the formula given for calculating the BMR of a woman rather than a man:
BMR= (10 x weight in kg) + (6.25 x height in cm) – (5 x age in years) -161
BMR = (10 x 80) + (6.25 x 170) – (5 x 32) – 161
BMR= 800 + 1062.5 -160 -161
The BMR of the woman in the question is therefore 1541.5 kcal

Question 18: D
This time, the information needs to be inserted into the formula for calculating the BMI of a man:
BMR= (10 x weight in kg) + (6.25 x height in cm) – (5 x age in years) + 5
BMR= (10 x 80) + (6.25 x 170) – (5 x 45) +5
BMR= 800 + 1062.5 -225 +5
The BMR of the man in the question is therefore 1642.5 kcal. The man does little to no exercise each week. It is therefore required to multiply 1642.5 by 1.2, which gives a daily recommended intake of 1971 kcal.

Question 19: C
It is easier to write out this calculation in the following format:
a b 7 –
  a b
———
5 6 5

From the above subtraction it is clear that b must be equal to 2 because 7 minus 2 is equal to 5, which is the unit term of the answer. It is now possible to rewrite the calculation with 2 substituted for b:
a 2 7 –
  a 2
———
5 6 5

From the above calculation it is possible to gauge certain facts. A must be greater than 5 because 1 is carried over to the second term:
a ^{1}2 7 –
  a 2
———
5 6 5

It is now clear than a must be equal to 6 because 12 minus 6 is equal to 6, which is the tens value of the answer.

ANSWERS MOCK PAPER C

Question 20: B
The mean is the sum of all of the numbers divided by the number of terms. From the information, we know that the sum of the first 8 numbers divided by 8 is equal to 44 plus the sum of the first 8 numbers all divided by 10. An expression for this can be written like this:

$$\frac{\text{sum of 8 numbers}}{8} = y = \frac{\text{sum of 8 numbers} + 44}{10}$$

Two equations can be derived from the above expression:

10y = sum of 8 numbers +44
8y = sum of 8 numbers

If we subtract the second equation from the first, we are left with: 2y=44 → y=22

The value of y and the average of both sets of numbers is therefore 22.

Question 21: D
There are three different options for staying at the hotel. They could either pay for three single rooms for £180, one single and one double room for £165, or one four-person room for £215.

Subtracting the cleaning cost for one night would leave:
£180-(3x£12) = £144
£165-(2x£12) = £141
£215-£12 = £203

The cheapest option is one single and one double room, and they want to stay three nights, which gives £141x3 = £423.

Question 22: C
Firstly, construct two algebraic equations: A-18=B-25 and $A=\frac{5}{6}B$

Solve these two equations as simultaneous equations by substituting $\frac{5}{6}B$ for A in equation 1:

$\frac{5}{6}$B-18=B-25

$7=\frac{1}{6}$B

B=42

Put B=42 back into equation 2: A= 42 x $\frac{5}{6}$

A=35

Question 23: C
Statement 1 is true. High temperatures and pH extremes cause a permanent alteration to the highly specific shape of the active site so that the substrate can no longer bind, and the enzyme no longer works.
Statement 2 is false. Amylase is produced in the salivary glands, pancreas, and small intestine.
Statement 3 is true.
Statement 4 is false. Bile is stored in the gall bladder, but it does travel down the bile duct to neutralise hydrochloric acid found in the stomach.
Statement 5 is true. Fructose is sweeter than glucose so smaller amounts can be used in food used in the slimming industry.

Question 24: C
The combining of food with bile and digestive enzymes occurs in the duodenum of the small intestine. In the ileum of the small intestine, the digested food is absorbed into the blood and lymph. The digested food then progresses into the large intestine. In the colon, water is reabsorbed. Faeces are then stored in the rectum and leave the alimentary canal via the anus.

Question 25: C
Statement 1 is true.
Statement 2 is true. For example, the drug curare, a South American plant toxin which is used in arrow poison, stops the nerve impulse from crossing the synapse and causes paralysis and can stop breathing.
Statement 3 is false. The sheath provides insulation for the nerve axon and increases the speed of impulse transmission via saltatory conduction.
Statement 4 is false. The peripheral nervous system includes motor and sensory neurons carrying impulses between receptors, effectors, and the central nervous system. The CNS consists of the spinal cord and the brain.
Statement 5 is true. A reflex arc travels from sensory neuron to relay neuron to motor neuron and is an innate mechanism designed to keep the animal safe. For example, it allows a person to quickly draw their hand away from a flame.

Question 26: D
Statement 1 is false because the pulmonary artery carries deoxygenated blood from the right ventricle to the lungs.
Statement 2 is true. This property of the aorta allows it to carry blood at high pressure and is why it pulsates.
Statement 3 is false because the mitral valve, otherwise known as the bicuspid valve, is between the left atrium and left ventricle.
Statement 4 is true.

Question 27: B
Statement 1 is true. Males have one X chromosome so if the allele is present they will be affected. Females have two X chromosomes so both need to be affected to be red-green colour blind as the condition is recessive
Statement 2 is true because according to the Punnett square below half of the children will have the homozygous recessive tt genotype and so will be non-rollers.

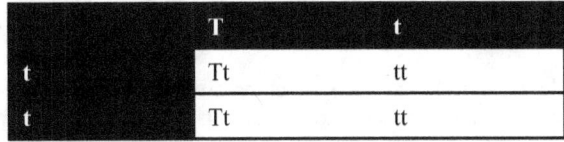

Statement 3 is true because all of the male children will inherit an X chromosome from the mother which will carry the colour-blind allele.

Question 28: E
Statement 1 is true.
Statement 2 is true. Decomposers in the soil break down urea and the bodies of dead organisms and this results in the production of ammonia in the soil.
Statement 3 is true.
Statement 4 is true.

ANSWERS MOCK PAPER C

Question 29: D
Statement 1 is false. Sucrose is a disaccharide formed by the condensation of two monosaccharides (glucose and fructose).
Statement 2 is false. Lactose is a disaccharide formed by condensation of a glucose molecule with a galactose molecule.
Statement 3 is true. Glucose has two isomers: alpha-glucose and beta-glucose.
Statement 4 is true.
Statement 5 is true.

Question 30: F
Alleles are different versions of the same gene. If you are a homozygous for a trait, you have two identical alleles for that particular gene, and if you are heterozygous you have two different alleles of that gene. Recessive traits only appear in the phenotype when there are no dominant alleles for that trait, i.e. two recessive alleles are carried.

Question 31: D
Remember that red blood cells don't have a nucleus and therefore have no DNA. In meiosis, a diploid cell divides in such a way so as to produce four haploid cells. Any type of cell division will require energy.

Question 32: C
The hypothalamus detects too little water in the blood, so the pituary gland releases ADH. The kidney maintains the blood water level, and allows less water to be lost in the urine until the blood water level returns to normal.

Question 33: E
Venous blood has a higher level of carbon dioxide and lower oxygen. Carbon dioxide forms carbonic acid in aqueous solution, thus making the pH of venous blood slightly more acidic than arterial blood. This leaves only E and F as possibilities, but releasing pH levels cannot fluctuate significantly gives pH 7.4.

Question 34: E
The cytoplasm is 80% water, but also contains, among other things, electrolytes and proteins. The cytoplasm doesn't contain everything, e.g. DNA is found in the nucleus.

Question 35: C
ATP is produced in mitochondria in aerobic respiration and in the cytoplasm during anaerobic respiration only.

Question 36: C
The cell membrane allows both active transport and passive transport by diffusion of certain ions and molecules, and is found in eukaryotes and prokaryotes like bacteria. It is a phospholipid bilayer.

Question 37: A
1 and 2 only: 223 PAIRS = 446 chromosomes; meiosis produces 4 daughter cells with half of the original number of chromosomes each, while mitosis produces two daughter cells with the original number of chromosomes each.

Question 38: E
If Bob is homozygous dominant (RR) the probability of having a child with red hair is 0%. However, if Bob is heterozygous (Rr), there is a 50% chance of having a child with red hair, since Mary must be homozygous recessive (rr) to have red hair. As we do not know Bob's genotype, both possibilities must be considered.

Question 39: A
If an offspring is born with red hair, it confirms Bob is heterozygous (Rr). He cannot have a red-haired child if he is homozygous dominant (RR), and would himself have red hair were he homozygous recessive (rr).

Question 40: A
Monohybrid cross rr and Rr results in 50% Rr and 50% rr offspring. 50% of offspring will have black hair, but they will be heterozygous for the hair allele.

Question 41: C
Statement 1 is true.
Statement 2 is false. The transition metals are both malleable and ductile, they conduct heat and electricity and they form positive ions when reacted with non-metals.
Statement 3 is true. Thermal decomposition is a reaction whereby a substance breaks down into two or more other substances due to heat. When a transition metal carbonate is heated, metal oxide and carbon dioxide are produced. The carbon dioxide can be collected and will turn limewater cloudy.
An example of this reaction is: $CuCO_3 \rightarrow CuO + CO_2$
Statement 4 is false. Transition metal hydroxides are insoluble in water.
Statement 5 is true.

Question 42: E
There are 9 Sulphur atoms on the left so there must be 9 on the right. Therefore, the values of B and C must add to make 9. This can be written as an equation: B+C=9
It is now useful to try to balance the Oxygen atoms: 4A+36 = 10+4B+4C+14
Simplify to give: 12 = 4B+4C-4A
Equation 1 can now be substituted into equation 2 to give: 12 = (4x9)-4A
24 = 4A →A = 6
There are 6 Potassium atoms on the left. This means that there must also be 6 potassium atoms on the right, so B must by 3. As shown in equation 1, B and C add to make 9 so C must be 6.

5 $PhCH_3$ + **6** $KMnO_4$ + **9** H_2SO_4 = **5** $PhCOOH$ + **3** K_2SO_4 + **6** $MnSO_4$ + **14** H_2O

Question 43: A
This question requires the use of the equation: $C = \frac{n}{v}$ where C= concentration, n= moles and v=volume
Convert 25cm³ into litres to get 0.025 litres and plug the values for concentration and volume into the equation to get the number of moles: $0.1 = \frac{n}{0.025}$ so n=0.0025
This question also requires the use of the equation: $n = \frac{m}{Mr}$ where m=mass, n=moles and Mr= molecular mass
The molecular mass is the sum of one calcium and two chlorine atoms which is equal to 111gmol⁻¹.
Inserting the molecular mass and number of moles into the above equation can be used to calculate the mass of calcium chloride: $m = 0.0025 \times 111 = 0.28g$

Question 44: E
This question requires use of the equation: Percentage yield = $\frac{actual\ yeild\ (g)}{predicted\ yield\ (g)}$ x 100.
If all of the benzene was converted to product (100 percent yield) then 20.5g of nitrobenzene would be produced:
13g C_6H_6 x $\frac{1\ mol\ C6H6}{78g\ C6H6}$ x $\frac{123g\ C6H5NO2}{1\ mol\ C6H5NO2}$ = 20.5g $C_6H_5NO_2$.
However, only 16.4g are actually produced. Using the equation, we can now calculate the percentage yield:
$\frac{16.4g}{20.5g}$ x 100 = 80% yield.

Question 45: E
The question is asking for which of the statements are *false*.
Statement 1 is true.
Statement 2 is true.
Statement 3 is false. Ionic compounds do conduct electricity when dissolved in water or when melted because the ions can move and carry current. On the other hand, solid ionic compounds do not conduct electricity.
Statement 4 is true. Alloys contain different sized atoms, making it harder for the layers of atoms to slide over each other.

ANSWERS MOCK PAPER C

Question 46: D
The Ar of Carbon is 12, Hydrogen is 1 and Oxygen is 16. Therefore, 12g of carbon is 1 mole of carbon; 2g of H is 2 moles of hydrogen and 16g of O is 1 mole of oxygen. The empirical formula is therefore CH_2O. The molecular weight is 30 g.mol^{-1}, which goes into 120 g.mol^{-1} exactly 4 times. The empirical formula must therefore be multiplied by 4 to obtain the molecular formula so the molecular formula is $C_4H_8O_4$.

Question 47: C
Statement 1 is true.
Statement 2 is false. The melting and boiling points increase as you go down the group.
Statement 3 is true.
Statement 4 is false. Chloride is more reactive than bromine, so no displacement reaction occurs.
Statement 5 is true.

Question 48: F
Ammonia is 1 nitrogen and 3 hydrogen atoms bonded covalently. N = 14g and H = 1g per mole, so percentage of N in NH_3 = 14g/17g = 82%. It can be produced from N_2 through fixation or the industrial Haber process for use in fertiliser, and may break down to its components.

Question 49: A
Milk is weakly acidic, pH 6.5-7.0, and contains fat. This is broken down by lipase to form fatty acids - turning the solution slightly more acidic.

Question 50: C
Glucose loses four hydrogen atoms; one definition of an oxidation reaction is a reaction in which there is loss of hydrogen.

Question 51: C
Isotopes have the same number of protons and electrons, but a different number of neutrons. The number of neutrons has no impact on the rate of reactions.

Question 52: E
$Mg + H_2SO_4 \rightarrow MgSO_4 + H_2$
Number of moles of Mg = $\frac{6}{24}$ = 0.25 moles.
1 mole of Mg reacts with 1 mole H_2SO_4 to produce 1 mole of magnesium sulphate. Therefore, 0.25 moles H_2SO_4 will react to produce 0.25 moles of $MgSO_4$.
M_r of H_2SO_4 = 2 + 32 + 64 = 98g per mole
The mass of H_2SO_4 used = 0.25 moles x 98g per mole = 24.5g.
Since 30g of H_2SO_4 is present, H_2SO_4 is in excess and the magnesium is the limiting reagent.
M_r of $MgSO_4$ = 24 + 32 + 64 = 120g per mole
The mass of $MgSO_4$ produced = 0.25 moles x 120g per mole = 30g which is the same mass as that of sulphuric acid in the original reaction.

Question 53: B
Start by multiplying each term by ax to give: $a(y+x)=x^2+a^2$
Expand the brackets: $ay+ax=x^2+a^2$
Subtract ax from both sides: $ay=x^2+a^2-ax$
Lastly, divide the both sides by a to get: $y = \frac{x^2+a^2-ax}{a}$

ANSWERS   MOCK PAPER C

Question 54: C
Solve as simultaneous equations. Start by substituting $x = \frac{y}{3}$ into equation B.
This gives $y = \frac{18}{y} - 7$
Multiply every term by y to give:
$0 = y^2 + 7y - 18$
Factorise this quadratic to give:
$0 = (y+9)(y-2)$
Where the graphs meet, y is equal to 2 and 9. Then y=3x so the graphs meet when x = 6 and x = 27

Question 55: B
To win one game, Rupert must win one squash game and one tennis game. In order to calculate the probability one winning one game, it is necessary to add the probability of winning one tennis game and losing one squash game to the probability of losing one tennis game and winning one squash game. The following calculation must be performed: $(\frac{3}{4} \times \frac{2}{3}) + (\frac{1}{4} \times \frac{1}{3}) = \frac{7}{12}$

Question 56: C
The numbers can all be written as a fraction over 36:

➢ $0.\dot{3}$ is the same as $\frac{12}{36}$
➢ $\frac{11}{18}$ is the same as $\frac{22}{36}$
➢ 0.25 is the same as $\frac{9}{36}$
➢ 0.75 is the same as $\frac{27}{36}$
➢ $\frac{62}{72}$ is the same as $\frac{31}{36}$
➢ $\frac{7}{7}$ is the same as $\frac{36}{36}$

Ordering them from lowest to highest gives: $\frac{7}{36}$; 0.25; $0.\dot{3}$; $\frac{11}{18}$; 0.75; $\frac{62}{72}$; $\frac{7}{7}$
Therefore, the median value is $\frac{11}{18}$

Question 57: B
This question requires the use of the equation:
p=mv where p=momentum, m=mass and v=velocity.

The total momentum before the collision is equal to the sum of the momentum of carriage 1 (12000 x 5) and carriage 2 (8000 x 0), which is 60,000 kg ms^{-1}. Momentum is conserved before and after the collision so the total momentum after the event also equal 60,000 kg ms^{-1}. The carriages now move together so the combined mass is 20,000kg. Using the equation again, the total momentum (60,000 kg ms^{-1}) divided by the total mass (20,000 kg) gives the velocity of the train carriages after the crash, which is equal to 3 ms^{-1}.

Question 58: C
Statement 1 is true.
Statement 2 is false because infrared has a longer wavelength than visible light.
Statement 3 is true.
Statement 4 is false because gamma radiation and not infrared radiation is used to sterilise food and to kill cancer cells.
Statement 5 is true because darker skins contain a higher amount of melanin pigment, which absorbs UV light.

Question 59: C
Statement 1 is false. In a nuclear reactor, every uranium nuclei split to release energy and three neutrons. An explosion could occur if all the neutrons are absorbed by further uranium nuclei as the reaction would escalate out of control. Control rods that are made of boron absorb some of the neutrons and control the chain reaction.
Statement 2 is false. Nuclear fusion occurs when a deuterium and tritium nucleus are forced together. The nuclei both carry a positive charge and consequently, very high temperatures and pressures are required to overcome the electrostatic repulsion. These temperatures and pressures are expensive and hard to repeat and so fusion is not currently suitable as a source of energy.
Statement 4 is true. During beta decay, a neutron transforms into a proton and an electron. The proton remains in the nucleus, whereas the electron is emitted and is referred to as a beta particle. The carbon-14 nucleus now has one more proton and one less neutron, so the atomic number increases by 1 and the atomic mass number remains the same.
Statement 5 is false. Beta particles are more ionising than gamma rays and less ionising than alpha particles.

Question 60: E
Firstly, deal with the term in the brackets: $3^3=27$
$(x^{½})^3 = x^{1.5}$
$(3x^{½})^3 = 27x^{1.5}$
Next, divide by $3x^2$: $\frac{27}{3} = 9$
$\frac{x^{1.5}}{x^2} = x^{-0.5} = \frac{1}{\sqrt{x}}$
Answer= $\frac{9}{\sqrt{x}}$

END OF PAPER

Mock Paper D Answers

Question 1: C
Mason and Dixon surveyed the North-eastern corner of the united states to end a border dispute. Symbolically, the line became the border between North and South in the dispute over slavery.

Question 2: D
Franz Kafka was a German-speaking Jew living in Prague.

Question 3: C
Mansa Musa ruled the Malian empire, whose gold mines made him absurdly wealthy.

Question 4: B
Japan occupied Manchuria, to universal outcry. In China, the invasion of Manchuria is considered to mark the beginnings of the Second World War.

Question 5: B
Isabella and Ferdinand united Spain through both their marriage, and by waging war on the Muslim population in the south. They finally took Grenada in 1492.

Question 6: A
The doppler effect.

Question 7: D
Hurricane Katrina hit Florida, Louisiana and the Gulf Coast, flooding large parts of New Orleans.

Question 8: A
Mens Rea is latin for guilty mind.

Question 9: C
China hosted the Olympics in Beijing in 2008, London, UK in 2012, and Rio de Jaineiro, Brazil in 2016. The 2020 Olympic Games will be held in Tokyo, Japan.

Question 10: B
Scientists cloned five identical monkeys. Monkeys have been cloned once before in 1999. Dolly, the first cloned sheep, was born in 1996 and Cows were first cloned in Japan in 1998.

Question 11: A
Cormac McCarthy, Thomas Pynchon and Toni Morrison are the only of those writers who are still alive.

Question 12: A
Although many of George Orwell's' writings deal with freedom and authority as themes, the word newspeak is only used in 1984 to denote the policing of language.

Question 13: C
The initial argument suggests that two things must be present for an action to happen. If only one is absent, the action cannot happen. Argument C has the same form, the others do not.

Question 14: E
Building model ships requires several positive traits. The passage does not tell us which the most important or most commonly lacked skill is, only that more than one skill is required for success.

ANSWERS MOCK PAPER D

Question 15: C
Joseph does not have blue cubic blocks, since all his blue blocks are cylindrical.

Question 16: B
The chance of red is 2/6 = 1/3. To get no reds at all, it must be non-red for each of three independent rolls. The probability of this is $(2/3)^3 = 8/27$. Therefore, the probability of at least one red is $1 – 8/27 = \underline{19/27}$

Question 17: D
These three furniture items are compatible with having 6 legs. All the other statements are false.

Question 18: D
Work this out by time. The friends are closing on each other at a total of 6mph overall, therefore the 42 miles take 7 hours. In seven hours, the falcon, flying at 18mph covers 18 x 7 = 126 miles.

Question 19: C
The passage tells us that antibiotic resistance could lead to people dying from Victorian diseases, and that liberal use of antibiotics in farming is the "most significant" contributor to this. Therefore it would be true to say that this use of antibiotics could cause serious harm.

Question 20: B
Calculate the overall cost of three stationery sets, then subtract any items not bought. For each item shared between two people, there is one of that item not required. The overall cost is £6.00 per person, £18.00 overall. Subtract one geometry set (£3), one paper pad (£1) and one pencil (50p) to give £13.50 overall cost.

Question 21: B
James runs 26.2 seconds, which is outside the qualifying time, therefore he does not qualify.

Question 22: A
Using s as the sandwich price, c for the crisps and w for the watermelon, the equation to solve is £5.60 $= s + c + w$.
Substituting in the information that $w = 2s$ and $s = 2c$:
£5.60 $= s + 2s + s/2$ or £5.60 $= 3.5 s$
$s = £1.60$
$Hence, w = 2 x £160 = £320$

Question 23: E
Haemoglobin is contained within red blood cells and is not free in the blood. Additionally, as a protein it is too large to normally pass through the glomerular filtration barrier. All the other substances are freely filtered.

Question 24: B
In order for the membrane potential to become more positive, there must be a net movement of positive ions into the muscle cell (so it becomes more positive compared to its resting state). Since there is a greater concentration of sodium ions outside, more sodium than potassium must move inwards.

Question 25: F
A polymer consists of repeating monomeric subunits. Polythene consists of multiple ethenes; glycogen of glucose; collagen of amino acids, starch of glucose; DNA of nucleotide bases, but triglycerides are not composed of monomeric subunits.

Question 26: E
Increased ADH causes more water reabsorption. This concentrates the sodium in the urine by reducing urine volume. In the healthy kidney, all glucose is reabsorbed and none is excreted into the urine.

ANSWERS — MOCK PAPER D

Question 27: D
Diastole is the relaxation phase of the cardiac cycle. In diastole the pressure in the aorta decreases as the contractile force from the ventricles is reduced. All of the other statements are true; the aortic valve closes after ventricular systole. All four chambers of the heart have blood in them throughout the cardiac cycle.

Question 28: B
Competitive inhibition occurs when the inhibitor prevents a reaction by binding to the enzyme active site. Hence, a higher concentration of the substrate can result in the same overall rate of reaction. i.e. the substrate outcompetes the competitor.

Non-competitive inhibition is where the inhibitor binds to the enzyme (not at the active site) and prevents the reaction from taking place. Increasing the substrate concentration therefore does not increase the reaction rate i.e. the substrate cannot outcompete the competitor as the enzymes are disabled and the competitor is not binding to the active site.

In this graph, line 1 shows the normal reaction without inhibition, line 2 shows competitive inhibitor and line 3 shows non-competitive inhibition.

Question 29: E
Nucleic acids are only found in the nucleus (DNA & RNA) and cytoplasm (RNA). They are not a component of the plasma membrane, whereas the other molecules are.

Question 30: D
The main artery to the lungs is the pulmonary artery, which gets blocked. The clot must therefore travel through the inferior vena cava and right side of the heart. It does not enter the superior vena cava or left (systemic) circulation.

Question 31: B
Note that the units are the same (M = moldm^{-3}), only the orders of magnitude are different. Convert the orders of magnitude to discover a 10^6 difference with more chloride than thyroxine

Question 32: B
Glycogen is not a hormone, it is a polysaccharide storage product primarily found in muscle and the liver.

Question 33: D
Reflexes can be influenced by the brain e.g. if you willingly pick up a hot plate, you will be able to withstand much greater heat than if you touch it by accident and discover it is hot. Reflex actions are fast as they usually bypass the brain. Since they are mediated by nerves, they are much faster than endocrine responses. Most animals show basic reflexes like the heat-withdrawal reflex which requires both sensory and motor components.

Question 34: D
The key here is to note that the answers are several orders of magnitude apart so you can round the numbers to make your calculations easier:
Probability of bacteria being resistant to every antibiotic =
P (Res to Antibiotic 1) x P (Res to Antibiotic 2) x P (Res to Antibiotic 3) x P (Res to Antibiotic 4)
$= \frac{100}{10^{11}} \times \frac{1000}{10^9} \times \frac{100}{10^8} \times \frac{1}{10^5}$
$= \frac{10^8}{10^{33}} = \frac{1}{10^{25}}$

Question 35: A
Producers are found at the bottom of food chains and always have the largest biomass.

Question 36: C
When the chest walls expand, the intra-thoracic pressure decreases. This causes the atmospheric pressure outside the chest to be greater than pressure inside the chest, resulting in a flow of air into the chest.

Question 37: F
All the statements are true; the carbon and nitrogen cycles are examinable in Section 2, so make sure you understand them! The atmosphere is 79% inert N_2 gas, which must be 'fixed' to useable forms by high-energy lightning strikes or by bacterial mediation. Humans also manually fix nitrogen for fertilisers with the Haber process.

Question 38: H
None of the above statements are correct. Mutations can be silent, cause a loss of function, or even a gain in function, depending on the exact location in the gene and the base affected. Mutations only cause a change in protein structure if the amino acids expressed by the gene affected are changed. This is normally due to a shift in reading frame. Whilst cancer arises as a result of a series of mutations, very few mutations actually lead to cancer.

Question 39: C
Remember that heart rate is controlled via the autonomic nervous system, which isn't a part of the central nervous system.

Question 40: H
None of the above are correct. There is no voluntary input to the heart in the form of a neuronal connection. Parasympathetic neurones slow the heart and sympathetic nervous input accelerates heart rate.

Question 41: C
It's important to know your reactivity series as its easy marks. Remember that potassium is more reactive than sodium, as it has a greater number of electron shells, with the outermost single electron being more loosely attracted to the nucleus because of this, and hence more likely to be lost. Following this pattern, sodium is the next most reactive and copper the least.

Question 42: E
144ml of water is 144g, which is the equivalent of 8 moles. 8 times Avogadro's constant gives the number of molecules present, which is 4.8×10^{24}. There are 10 protons and 10 electrons in each water molecule, hence there are 4.8×10^{25} electrons.

Question 43: F
Write the equation to calculate molar ratios:
$C_8H_{18} + 12.5\ O_2 \rightarrow 8CO_2 + 9H_2O$
Travelling 10 miles uses: 228 x 10 = 2,280g of Octane.
M_r of Octane = 12 x 8 + 18 x 1 = 114
Number of moles of octane used = 2,280/114 = 20 moles. Thus, 160 moles of CO_2 must be produced.
M_r of CO_2 = 12 + 16 x 2 = 44
Mass of CO_2 produced = 44 x 160 = 7,040 g = 7.04 kg

Question 44: F
Reactivity series of metals:
Cu is more reactive than Ag and will displace it.
Ca is more reactive than H and will displace it.
2 and 4 are incorrect because Fe is higher in the reactivity series than Cu and Fe is lower in the reactivity series than Ca, so no displacement will occur.

Question 45: G
Moving left to right is the equivalent of moving down the metal reactivity series (i.e. Na is most reactive and Zn is least reactive). Therefore, moving from left to right, the reactivity of the metals decreases, likelihood of corrosion decreases, less energy is required to separate metals from their ores and metals lose electrons less readily to form positive ions.

ANSWERS — MOCK PAPER D

Question 46: F
Halogens become less reactive as you progress down group 17. Thus in order of increasing reactivity from left to right: I→ Br→ Cl. Therefore, I will not displace Br, Cl will displace Br and Br will displace I.

Question 47: A
Wires are made out of copper because it is a good conductor of electricity. Copper is also used in coins (not aluminium). Aluminium is resistant to corrosion but because of a layer of aluminium oxide (not hydroxide).

Question 48: C
$2Li + 2H_2O \rightarrow 2LiOH + H_2$
Therefore, 2 moles of Li react to produce 1 mole of H_2 gas (24 dm^3).
The number of moles of Li = $\frac{21}{7}$ = 3 moles.
Thus, 1.5 moles of H_2 gas are produced = 36 dm^3.

Question 49: B
$MgCl_2$ contains stronger bonds than NaCl because Mg ions have a 2+ charge, thus having a stronger electrostatic pull for negative chloride ions. The smaller atomic radius also means that the nucleus has less distance between it and incoming electrons. Transition metals are able to form multiple stable ions e.g. Fe^{2+} and Fe^{3+}.

Covalently bonded structures do tend to have lower MPs than ionically bonded, but the giant covalent structures (diamond and graphite for example) have very high melting points. Graphite is an example of a covalently bonded structure which conducts electricity.

Question 50: D
Energy is released from reaction **A**, as shown by a negative enthalpy. The reaction is therefore exothermic. Since energy is released, the product CO_2 has less energy than the reactants did. Therefore, CO_2 is more stable. Reaction **B** has a positive enthalpy, which means energy must be put into the reaction for it to occur i.e. it's an endothermic reaction. That means that the products (CaO and CO_2) have more energy and are less stable than the reactants ($CaCO_3$).

Question 51: B
Solid oxides are unable to conduct electricity because the ions are immobile. Metals are extracted from their molten ores by electrolysis. Fractional distillation is used to separate miscible liquids with similar boiling points. Mg^{2+} ions have a greater positive charge and a smaller ionic radius than Na^+ ions, and therefore have stronger bonds.

Question 52: E
Li^+ (2) and Na^+ (2, 8)
Mg^{2+} (2, 8) and Ne (2, 8)
Na^{2+} (2, 7) and Ne (2, 8)
O^{2-} (2, 4) and a Carbon atom (2, 4)

Question 53: B
Equate the volume with the surface area in the proportion instructed by the question. $3(^4/_3\pi r^3) = 4\pi r^2$, simplifies to r = 1.

Question 54: B
Gravitational potential energy increases as the grain is lifted further from floor; this is equal to the work done against gravity to attain the higher position. The potential energy equal to mgΔh, so it is dependent upon the mass of the grain that is lifted.

Question 55: E
This is a tricky question that requires a conceptual leap. Only the top candidates will get this correct.
Surface Area of Earth $= 4\pi r^2$
$= 4 \times 3 \times (0.6 \times 10^7)^2$
$= 12 \times (6 \times 10^6)^2$
$= 12 \times 36 \times 10^{12}$
$= 3.6 \times 10^{14}$

Since $= \frac{Force}{Area}$, $Atmospheric\ Pressure = \frac{Force\ exerted\ by\ atmosphere}{Surface\ Area\ of\ Earth}$
Therefore: $Force = 10^5 \times 3.6 \times 10^{14} = 3.6 \times 10^{19}\ N$

The force exerted by the atmosphere is equal to its weight therefore:
$Force = Weight = mass \times g$
Hence, $Atmospheric\ Mass = \frac{3.6 \times 10^{19}}{10} = 3.6 \times 10^{18}\ Kg$

Question 56: D
F = ma; therefore the difference in force is equal to $m_1 a_1 - m_2 a_2$. This equals (6 x 6) – (2 x 8) = 20N

Question 57: B
Number of annual flights = Flights per hour x Number of hours in one year x Number of airports
$= 4 \times (24 \times 365) \times 1000 = 96 \times 365 \times (1000) \approx 100 \times 365 \times 10 \times 100 = 365 \times 10^5 = 36.5\ Million$

However, this is an overestimate since we have multiplied by 100 instead of 96. Hence, the actual answer will be slightly lower. 35 Million is the only other viable option available.
365x24=8760 is the number of hours in a year, then 8760 x number of flights per hour (4) = 35040 flights per year per airport. Multiply by the number of airports – 42 million to the nearest million.

Question 58: A
Because the two sides of the circuit are in parallel, both sets of lights experience a 24v voltage drop across them. In lights R and S this is shared equally between them, but in lights P and Q, the new light with twice the resistance takes twice the voltage in accordance with Ohm's Law (V= IR).

Question 59: D
Add the first and last equations together to give: 2F = 4, thus F = 2.
Then add the second and third equations to give 2F – 2H= 5. Thus, H = -0.5
Finally, substitute back in to the first equation to give 2 + G – 0.5 = 1. Thus, G = -0.5
Therefore, FGH = 2 x -0.5 x -0.5 = 0.5.

Question 60: E
This is a simple recall question. X rays have the shortest wavelength whilst microwaves have the longest wavelengths with visible light being somewhere in the middle. It is well worth your time remembering the basic positions of the components of the electromagnetic spectrum as it frequently gets tested in the IMAT.

END OF PAPER

FINAL ADVICE

Arrive well rested, well fed and well hydrated

The IMAT is an intensive test, so make sure you're ready for it. Unlike the UKCAT, you'll have to sit this at a fixed time (normally at 9AM). Thus, ensure you get a good night's sleep before the exam (there is little point cramming) and don't miss breakfast. If you're taking water into the exam then make sure you've been to the toilet before so you don't have to leave during the exam. Make sure you're well rested and fed in order to be at your best!

Move on

If you're struggling, move on. Every question has equal weighting and there is no negative marking. In the time it takes to answer on hard question, you could gain three times the marks by answering the easier ones. Be smart to score points- especially in section two where some questions are far easier than others.

Make Notes on your Essay

Some universities may ask you questions on your IMAT essay at the interview. Sometimes you may have the interview as late as March which means that you **MUST** make short notes on the essay title and your main arguments after the essay. This is especially important if you're applying to UCL and Cambridge where the essay is discussed more frequently.

Afterword

Remember that the route to a high score is your approach and practice. Don't fall into the trap that *"you can't prepare for the IMAT"* – this could not be further from the truth. With knowledge of the test, some useful time-saving techniques and plenty of practice you can dramatically boost your score.

Work hard, never give up and do yourself justice.

Good Luck!

Acknowledgements

I would like to thank the UniAdmissions Tutors for all their hard work and advice in compiling this book.

Alex

About Us

Infinity Books is the publishing division of *Infinity Education Ltd*. We currently publish over 85 titles across a range of subject areas – covering specialised admissions tests, examination techniques, personal statement guides, plus everything else you need to improve your chances of getting on to competitive courses such as medicine and law, as well as into universities such as Oxford and Cambridge.

Outside of publishing we also operate a highly successful tuition division, called UniAdmissions. This company was founded in 2013 by Dr Rohan Agarwal and Dr David Salt, both Cambridge Medical graduates with several years of tutoring experience. Since then, every year, hundreds of applicants and schools work with us on our programmes. Through the programmes we offer, we deliver expert tuition, exclusive course places, online courses, best-selling textbooks and much more.

With a team of over 1,000 Oxbridge tutors and a proven track record, UniAdmissions have quickly become the UK's number one admissions company.

Visit and engage with us at:

Website (Infinity Books): www.infinitybooks.co.uk

Website (UniAdmissions): www.uniadmissions.co.uk

Facebook: www.facebook.com/uniadmissionsuk

Twitter: @infinitybooks7